MY OTHER E

QUICK AND DIRTY TIPS FOR SURVIVING AN ILEOSTOMY

AW CROSS

GLORY BOX PRESS

My Other Bag's a Prada: Quick and Dirty Tips for Surviving an Ileostomy

Cover illustration by Peter Cross
Cover design by germancreative
Book design and production by Glory Box Press
Editing by Mia Darien

AW Cross
gloryboxpress.com
contact@gloryboxpress.com

Printed in Canada

First Printing: July 2016

ISBN 978-0-9950991-3-5

ABOUT THE AUTHOR

A.W. Cross is a Canadian author and blogger. She has experienced the entire gamut of ulcerative colitis from diagnosis to j-pouch, including an intense love/hate relationship with her ostomy, Lips. Whenever she has time, she enjoys her family, friends, and video games.

You can follow her on Twitter @ScreamingMeemi or visit her blog, screamingmeemie.com

My Other Bag's a Prada: Quick and Dirty Tips for Surviving an Ileostomy is her second book.

Other titles in the *Quick and Dirty Tips for Surviving* Series:

You Don't Look Sick: Quick and Dirty Tips for Surviving Ulcerative Colitis
Unicorn Farts and Glitter: Quick and Dirty Tips for Surviving a J-Pouch

For all ostomates: may your blow-outs be few and pancakes something you eat for breakfast.

CONTENTS

PREFACE

I was diagnosed with ulcerative colitis in 2009. My condition deteriorated over the next few years until I finally had my colon removed in 2011. Having a colectomy was the best thing that could have happened to me. I knew I was ill, but I didn't realize just *how* ill I was until I got my ileostomy. The idea of a stoma is a source of fear for many people, but I can say, wholeheartedly and with all the cliché of truth, that having the operation gave me my life back.

My stoma was not a perfect fix; far from it. There were many bleak moments during my time as an ostomate: blow-outs, obstructions, and my skin literally peeling off before my eyes. But the worst part was that most non-medical ostomy discussions—usually by fellow ostomates—painted a very grim picture of my situation. I was terrified.

But I was also lucky: not too long after I had my surgery, I found a person whose levity about our shared circumstances bordered on the scandalous. And then another. And another. And, as when I had ulcerative colitis, being able to find humor in even my lowest moments was the silver lining I needed to get me through.

In 2015 (now sans ostomy), I joined the NaNoWriMo rebellion and wrote what would eventually become three books; this is the second. Writing about what I learned during my illness also inspired me to create my IBD blog, screamingmeemie.com.

I hope this book saves you some trouble, and I hope it makes you smile—even just once.

AW Cross, 2016

INTRODUCTION

It may be that your inflammatory bowel disease went refractory. Perhaps you developed cancer or an increased risk of it. Possibly you were injured, or you suffered from incontinence or an obstruction. Whatever the reason, the scourge of whatever plagued your body and ruined your colon has been dealt a mortal blow. You had your colon removed; you have an ileostomy.

You may have won that battle, but the war is in no way over. You're now an ostomate. You need a whole new combat plan: you must choose your appliance wisely, remain vigilant against , blow-outs, and obstructions, and most important, have the confidence to cope successfully every day.

Within these pages is your new arsenal: quick and dirty tips for successfully coping with an ileostomy. You'll learn the basics of choosing an appliance, dealing with leaks and odor, and what to pack in your survival kit. You'll discover strategies for dealing with the physical and emotional consequences of your new body, and you'll be drilled in the finer points of hospital etiquette, ostomy fashion, and the bewilderment of the common man.

This book contains little medical advice; it is a practical guide to living daily with an ileostomy. Gleaned from personal experience, the information contained herein is the result of numerous successes and failures. Whether your stoma is temporary or permanent, the methods are the same.

This book will not change your bag for you, but it will save you time, pain, and your sanity.

ILEOSTOMY

MY OTHER BAG'S A PRADA

DISADVANTAGES OF AN ILEOSTOMY

You've probably figured out that now that you no longer have a colon, life is pretty sweet. And it is, most of the time. But what good is sweet without any sour?

First, the not-so-sweet side of having an ileostomy:

YOU NO LONGER GET TO FART IN THE TRADITIONAL WAY
This may not seem like a big deal at first, but trust me, you'll miss it.

POUCHES CAN BE AWKWARD
At first. You'll learn to love/hate it.

ACCIDENTS WILL HAPPEN
It's a given; no need to cry over spilled poop.

YOU MAY GET BLOCKAGES
Know the signs, get it sorted.

YOU'RE A MYSTERY
Since having an ostomy is somewhat uncommon, there is a lack of knowledge among general healthcare providers about

treatment when things go wrong.

YOUR BODY IMAGE MAY SUFFER
You may find the idea of a stoma and an external bag disconcerting.

IT'S NOT FOR THE SQUEAMISH
Part of your intestine is now outside of your body, AND you're pooping from your front instead of your back . . . into a bag you have to empty by hand.

YOUR SKIN GETS DAMAGED EASILY
You no longer have the bulk in your stool to absorb all your digestive enzymes; where those enzymes touch, burning ensues.

ADVANTAGES OF AN ILEOSTOMY

But when it's sweet, it's super-sweet:

NO MORE ULCERATIVE COLITIS/BOWEL CANCER/ FAMILIAL ADENOMATOUS POLYPOSIS/WHATEVER!
Woot! You're freeeeeeeeee.

YOU'LL TAKE FEWER MEDICATIONS
Goodbye, steroids and foam enemas!

YOU'LL HAVE LESS PAIN
No more colon to make those awful, gut-wrenching cramps.

YOUR POUCH LOOKS LIKE SCIENCE-FICTION BAD-ASSERY
You are a hardcore miracle of medical science.

NO MORE DIARRHEA
Well, not from your butt, anyway.

YOU CAN 'BURP' YOUR BAG
Instant sneak attack and conversation stopper.

IT'S PRACTICALLY A NEW ACCESSORY
One-piece, two-piece, closed, drainable, transparent, opaque. So many choices!

YOU CAN EAT SPICY FOOD WITHOUT FEAR OF REPERCUSSIONS
Glorious, mouth-burning, lip-shriveling spicy food.

SMALL CHILDREN THINK YOU'RE SUPER-COOL OR SUPER-SCARY
Either way, it's a win.

IT'S LIKELY NOT AS BAD AS YOU THOUGHT IT WOULD BE
Once you get your head around it, it will all seem very normal.

DISCONNECTED

PHYSICAL CONSEQUENCES OF AN ILEOSTOMY

PHYSICAL CONSEQUENCES OF AN ILEOSTOMY AND HOW TO COPE

Obviously, the biggest physical change that you will undergo is having your colon removed and a stoma created. You may have an endostomy or a loop ostomy; it may be permanent or temporary; your stoma may protrude, retract, or sit right where you want it. No matter what kind of stoma you have, there are common physical side effects that you will likely experience as an ostomate:

FATIGUE

Some ostomates find they become tired more quickly; others find they have an abundance of energy.

PAIN

Your surgical pain will improve after about six weeks, but you may find the area around your stoma remains tender.

ITCHINESS

The skin around your stoma (peristomal skin) will itch as it heals and as your body adjusts to your appliance. After you've healed, itchiness is caused by skin irritation.

SKIN IRRITATION

Both your stomal and peristomal skin can become irritated by your ostomy appliance and by frequent or prolonged contact with your stoma output. Skin irritation can become severe if left untreated.

NAUSEA

Any nausea should improve as your body adjusts to its changes.

B12 DEFICIENCY

B12 deficiency can be difficult to recognize; certain symptoms, such as fatigue and loss of appetite, are general, and other symptoms can mimic dehydration. If you begin experiencing nerve and vision disturbances, have your B12 checked.

WEIGHT FLUCTUATIONS

You may lose weight because you struggle to eat as much as you should, or you may gain weight because you can eat more than when you were ill.

DEHYDRATION

Since your colon is gone, it is absorbing even less water than when it was inflamed, increasing your risk of.

MUCUS

For the first week or two, you may find you have mucus drainage from your rectal stump.

PHANTOM RECTUM

You may feel as though your rectum is still intact, and that it wants to go to the bathroom. (And no, that mucus isn't ectoplasm.)

FEELING BETTER

Even with the long recovery from surgery and adjusting to your new pouch, now that the main site of your illness is gone, you'll probably feel much better.

POTENTIAL COMPLICATIONS

Some ostomates experience a litany of complications; others have none. Be aware of the following complications, and seek medical help accordingly:

NECROTIC STOMA
Your stoma will become discolored, turning from dark pink to purple, dark red, or black; it may also become dry and develop an odor. Sto000mal necrosis is caused by a lack of blood supply to your stoma.

MUCOCUTANEOUS SEPARATION
Mucocutaneous separation occurs when your peristomal skin separates from your stoma; you will be able to see a gap between the stoma and the edge of your skin. Separation of your peristomal skin can be caused by malnutrition (which affects your ability to heal), infection, steroid therapy, diabetes, or localized radiation.

STOMA PROLAPSE
Your stoma can become displaced and protrude further than normal. A prolapse can be caused by improper suturing of your stoma to your abdominal wall, a hole in your abdominal wall that is too large for your stoma, intense abdominal pressure, reduced muscle support, obesity, or pregnancy.

HERNIATED STOMA
Due to weakness in your abdominal wall, your bowel can protrude; the area around your stoma will bulge. can occur if you are overweight, lift heavy objects too soon after surgery, have extensive steroid therapy, or suffer a chronic cough.

OBSTRUCTION
Your stoma may become blocked and unable to pass stool. Obstructions are usually caused by strictures or food.

STOMA RETRACTION
Your stoma can retract below the surface of your skin, resulting in concave peristomal skin. Stoma retraction can be caused by factors including poor blood flow, obesity, malnutrition, and stenosis of your intestine.

ILEUS
Your bowel may become unable to move stool. Ileus is caused by an obstruction or temporary paralysis after surgery.

FISTULAS
Fistulas occur when channels form between your organs, or between the inside and outside of your body, such as through your abdominal wall. Fistulas are caused by inflammation and infection.

STOMA TRAUMA
Your stoma can be injured by physical trauma, by your clothing or by the appliance itself. A small amount of bleeding from the mucosal surface of your stoma is normal, but significant bleeding or any visible damage, such as a cut or ulceration, needs to be evaluated by a doctor.

TIPS FOR COPING

BE AWARE
Know which physical changes are normal and which are serious.

DON'T DELAY MEDICAL CARE
If you believe you have a complication, immediately contact your doctor or WOC (Wound, Ostomy, Continence)/ET (Enterostomal)/ostomy nurse. Ostomy complications can become serious very quickly.

TAKE YOUR MULTI-VITAMINS
Try to prevent any vitamin or mineral deficiencies.

ENSURE THAT YOUR MEDICATIONS, INCLUDING VITAMINS, WILL BE ABSORBED

Avoid sustained-release formulas, crush your tablets (check with your pharmacist first), or take liquid, gel caps, or gummy formulations. Remind your doctor to compensate for reduced transit times when they are prescribing medications. If you are unsure whether or not a medication will absorb in time, place one tablet in a glass of warm water for 30 minutes and see whether it dissolves.

MAINTAIN YOUR SKIN INTEGRITY

Change your appliance as often as you should, and treat any skin trouble as soon as it arises. Good hygiene is essential.

EAT A BALANCED DIET

Start with reliable, low-risk foods and gradually progress your diet to determine what foods you'll be able to cope with. Chew everything well.

EAT SALTIER FOODS

You will need extra salt for a few weeks until your body adjusts to your stoma.

STAY HYDRATED

Dehydration is annoying and uncomfortable at best, very serious at worst.

RELAX

Avoid significant physical activity for eight weeks after surgery, then increase your activity level gradually.

EXERCISE MODESTLY

Especially for the first three months. When you begin, start slow.

AVOID LIFTING

Don't lift anything remotely heavy for the first three months. After that, wear a support garment when you are lifting anything heavier than 10 pounds.

KEEP A JOURNAL

A journal will help you track your progress, which can be helpful if you have problems with your ostomy. Regularly charting how you feel will make it easier to spot patterns between good and bad days.

WEAR A PAD

If you have temporary rectal drainage, wear a pad or panty liner to absorb the waste.

HUMOR YOUR PHANTOM RECTUM

Sit on the toilet for a few minutes. Eventually, it will pass.

PROTECT YOUR STOMA

If you are playing contact sports or performing extreme physical activities, make sure your stoma is secure and covered with a stoma guard.

CAN'T WAIT: ACCESS TO PUBLIC BATHROOMS

Although knowledge about ostomies is increasing, the public services that support them vary between countries.

Through Crohn's and Colitis UK, ostomates are eligible for a *Can't Wait Card*, a wallet-size card which indicates the holder has a medical condition resulting in an urgency to use the bathroom. The cards encourage businesses to grant the holder access to washrooms that may not be available to the general public. Also available for UK patients is the *RADAR* key. Produced by the National Key Scheme, the key can be used to unlock public bathrooms all over the UK.

Crohn's and Colitis Australia also supports a *Can't Wait* program, which supplies cards to patient members, and *Can't Wait* stickers to businesses and retailers who will display the stickers in their windows, indicating to cardholders that their toilets are available when needed. *Can't Wait Cards* are also available in the United States through the Crohn's and Colitis Foundation of America.

At the time of writing, Canada's Can't Wait program is still in its infancy. Services currently available include the *GoHere Washroom Finder App*, which uses GPS to locate washrooms nearby and which can also be used to map out locations along a route of travel. There currently is no physical Can't Wait Card in Canada, but a virtual *GoHere Washroom Access Card* is available via the *Washroom Finder* app. A *GoHere* decal, similar to Australia's Can't Wait sticker, is also being trialed in several Canadian cities, with plans to go nationwide if the pilot is successful.

PAPA'S GOT A BRAND-NEW BAG

CHOOSING YOUR APPLIANCE AND ACCESSORIES

CHOOSING YOUR APPLIANCE

When you leave the hospital after your surgery, you'll be given a small supply of the ostomy appliance you wore during your stay, but it may not be a system that you want to use long-term. Fortunately, there are a variety of pouching systems from which to choose. The best way to determine which ostomy system works for you is through trial and error, and ostomy supply companies are more than happy to help by providing free samples of their various products. Take advantage of this generosity; you may have your ostomy for a long time, and you need to be as comfortable as possible to cope successfully. The choice can seem overwhelming at first; however, this 'pick n' mix' availability means you can create a system tailored to your specific needs.

A successful pouching system will:
- be easy to apply and remove
- allow you to obtain a good seal and prevent leaks
- not irritate your skin
- prevent odor

- last as long as intended by the manufacturer
- not be noticeable under your clothes
- be cost-effective

CHOOSING AN OSTOMY SYSTEM: PROS AND CONS

First, a quick glossary of terms:

Wafer: Also known as a skin barrier; the part of the appliance that sticks to your skin.

Bag/pouch: The bag attached to the wafer; collects your output/waste.

Flange: On a two-piece system, the plastic ring that connects the pouch to the wafer.

APPLIANCE OPTIONS
- one piece vs. two piece
- closed pouch vs. drainable pouch
- translucent vs. opaque
- filtered vs. non-filtered
- pre-cut vs. cut-to-fit vs. moldable skin barriers
- size (mini to extra-large to overnight pouches)
- normal vs. extended-wear wafers
- special requirements: convex wafer and stoma collars

You can mix and match all of these options to create a system that perfectly fits your needs.

ONE-PIECE VS. TWO-PIECE SYSTEM

ONE-PIECE SYSTEM
A one-piece system consists of a pouch fused to a wafer.

Pros:

- The pouch cannot become detached from the wafer.
- One-piece systems tend to be less bulky than two-piece systems.
- The flange is more flexible, which can help the appliance better adhere to scarred or otherwise uneven skin.
- One-piece systems are usually less expensive per unit than two-piece systems.

Cons:

- A one-piece must be changed more often than a two-piece system, which can be frustrating if you struggle to get a secure seal.
- Because you have to change your appliance more frequently, your skin is more likely to become irritated.
- One-piece systems are non-burp-able. ('Burping' is when you separate the top of the bag and the flange briefly to release gas and prevent your bag from bloating.)
- If used in conjunction with a closed bag, you'll have to change your entire appliance multiple times a day.

TWO-PIECE SYSTEM

A two-piece system consists of a wafer with a flange and a pouch with a connecting flange. When you are using a two-piece system, you must ensure that the size of the flange on the wafer and the size of the flange on the pouch are the same so that they fit together securely.

Pros:

- If your seal is good, the wafer can remain in place for up to a week. Not disturbing the wafer can reduce skin irritation.
- Changing your appliance less often reduces the number of times you have to try to get a good seal.
- Since you can put the wafer on before the pouch, it can be easier for you to position the appliance correctly, and allows you to more easily find and repair any gaps.

- There are both "clip on" and "stick on" flange systems available, providing more options for you if you have reduced manual dexterity.
- The bag can be "burped" to get rid of excess gas.

Cons:

- When applying the two pieces separately, you must work quickly; place gauze over your stoma to prevent waste getting into the flange.
- If waste does get into the flange, the connection is no longer secure and can result in leaks and odor. Your appliance must then either be thoroughly cleaned and dried or discarded.
- You may not notice leakage behind your flange until it causes skin irritation.
- Some two-piece systems are fairly bulky and may be uncomfortable under your clothes.
- The flange can be quite rigid, making it difficult to get a good seal if your skin is uneven.
- Two-piece systems are usually more expensive per unit than one-piece systems.

CLOSED VS. DRAINABLE POUCHES

CLOSED POUCH

A closed pouch has no drainage outlet, meaning that the pouch is usually discarded rather than emptied. Alternatively, you can insert a disposable pouch liner, allowing you to use the pouch multiple times.

Pros:

- When the pouch is full, you can just remove and throw it away; there's no need to drain it.
- If you use pouch liners, you can reuse the pouch.
- You have a fresh pouch multiple times a day.

- Closed pouches are more convenient for bulky output; the bag can just be disposed of rather than emptied.
- Both flushable pouches and liners are available, making disposal even easier.
- Since they lack a closure, closed pouches can be a more discreet option during intimacy.

Cons:

- If you have frequent output and are discarding your pouches, you may find the number of bags needed becomes costly.
- You may find it awkward to dispose of the bag when you are not at home.
- Emptying the bag before disposing of it can be tricky.

DRAINABLE POUCH

A drainable pouch has an opening at the bottom that allows it to be emptied without detaching it from the flange; the bag is then resealed and used again. The pouch is kept closed with a clip, a rolled Velcro® closure, or a spigot/valve.

Pros:

- The bag can be used up to three or four days, meaning you can change it less often.
- You use fewer pouches, which can be more cost-effective.
- Drainable bags are more efficient than closed systems if you have a lot of liquid output. Bags with the spigot or valve closure are especially helpful with high volumes of liquid waste.
- Pouches can be rinsed (or not) and then reattached.

Cons:

- The clip may occasionally come undone, especially if your bag is too full, or if the clip catches on your clothing. Rarely do the rolled Velcro®-systems come undone; accidents can usually be avoided by keeping the drainage outlet clean, and by emptying your bag before it gets too full.

- The clip, and sometimes even the Velcro®, can rub against your thigh and become irritating. Fix this by repositioning your pouch.
- If your output is very thick, draining your pouch can be like trying to squeeze a pastry bag; add a little water to loosen things up.

COLOR (TRANSLUCENT VS. OPAQUE)

Sadly, a choice of color does not mean a choice between leopard print and palm trees. Only children get a choice of patterned ostomy bags, an injustice which is only surpassed by the fact that any child should have to worry about an ostomy bag in the first place. Instead, color means a choice between translucent or opaque (flesh-toned or white).

TRANSLUCENT

Pros:

- A translucent bag makes it easy to monitor your output.
- Increased visibility also helps you keep tabs on your stoma.
- If you are using a one-piece or attaching your two-piece as a whole, a clear bag can make attaching your appliance easier, since you can see where the wafer is placed around your stoma; it can also help you identify and monitor leaks more quickly.
- Clear bags are often helpful for new ostomates, and likely what you will use in the hospital for the first few days.

Cons:

- Your waste is visible, which you may find unpleasant.

OPAQUE

Pros:

- If you aren't interested in watching your output or your stoma, you don't have to.
- Many ostomates feel it minimizes the psychological impact of having an ostomy.
- An opaque pouch is more discreet than a translucent pouch.

Cons:

- You may not notice a leak until it starts to burn.
- You may find it tricky to position a one-piece appliance correctly over your stoma, especially if you are a new ostomate. You may need several attempts per application.

FILTERED VS. NON-FILTERED POUCHES

FILTERED

The purpose of a pouch filter is to release excess gas from your pouch without any odor.

Pros:

- Since the filter releases excess gas from your pouch, you will need to burp your bag less often.
- The gas released has very little odor.

Cons:

- Filters tend to work better if your output is neither very bulky or very liquid; both tend to saturate the filter and clog it.
- If the filter becomes saturated, it can leak.
- The filter can become clogged after several days, even if output is moderate.
- A filter does not release all gas; sometimes burping is still necessary.

- The filter must be covered if there is a chance it will get wet, such as during swimming or showering. Stickers are provided with filtered pouches for this purpose.

NON-FILTERED POUCHES

Pros:

- You don't have to worry about covering a filter when you swim or have a shower.
- You don't have to worry about a filter becoming clogged or leaking.

Cons:

- You'll have to burp your bag to get rid of any excess gas.
- There can be a strong odor associated with burping.

PRE-CUT VS. CUT-TO-FIT VS. MOLDABLE SKIN BARRIERS

Your stoma will change size and even shape over time, especially in the months just after surgery. Ensuring that your skin barrier fits properly over your stoma is crucial to preventing your output from touching and degrading your skin over time.

PRE-CUT SKIN BARRIERS

In a pre-cut skin barrier, the stoma panel (the center portion of the barrier that fits around your stoma) has already been cut to a standard size. A pre-cut skin barrier is recommended only if your stoma has a consistent size and a regular, round shape.

Pros:

- If your stoma is a consistent size and shape, pre-cut wafers save you the time and hassle of measuring and cutting or molding to fit.

Cons:

- Your stoma size and shape must be consistent to ensure a good seal.

CUT-TO-FIT SKIN BARRIERS

Cut-to-fit wafers have a series of radial measurements printed on the stoma panel. Included in the box is a measurement guide, which you hold over your stoma to determine its current size. You then cut the panel to the precise measurement of your stoma.

Pros:

- If the size of your stoma fluctuates, you can cut your supplies as needed.

Cons:

- Cut-to-fit barriers are not recommended for stomas that have an irregular shape, as the panel can be tricky to cut appropriately.
- Measuring and cutting the stoma panel can be tedious and inconvenient.

MOLDABLE SKIN BARRIERS

A moldable wafer has a stoma panel that is placed over your stoma and molded into the correct size and shape.

Pros:

- You get a customized fit, which is ideal for stomas that may change in size or have an irregular shape. Also great for stomas that don't.

Cons:

- None.

POUCH SIZE

Ostomy bags come in a variety of sizes, and although you'll likely settle on a single size for everyday use, there are occasions where you'll find that a smaller or larger size is more appropriate. Each ostomy supply company tends to have their own range of sizes, and these sizes can also vary between the company's individual systems. In general, ostomy bag sizes include:

MINI (STOMA CAP)
Stoma caps are tiny, closed pouches intended for use during a time when your stoma is not very active since they hold a minimal amount of waste. Some ostomates use them while they irrigate their Kock pouch, but you can also use them for other short periods of time, such as during sex, or if you want to keep your stoma covered while you have a bath or go swimming. Stoma caps can also be used to cover mucous fistulas.

MINI (REGULAR POUCH)
Mini pouches tend to be approximately 4 ¾ inches to 6 inches in length. Mini pouches are a good option when you need a more discrete pouch, such as during intimacy, exercise, or if you're playing sports. Although they have a larger capacity than a stoma cap, mini pouches are intended for short-term use only. Mini pouches are not recommended if you have a high volume of liquid output.

SMALL
Small pouches are larger than mini pouches, ranging from approximately 7 to 10 inches in length. Since they hold a greater volume of output than a mini pouch, they can be worn for a longer period. Like mini pouches, small pouches are not a good choice if you have a lot of liquid output.

MEDIUM OR "STANDARD"
Standard-sized bags tend to be around 12 inches long; they are the most common pouch choice for regular wear, as they strike a balance

between discretion and capacity. Medium bags usually need to be emptied every few hours and are appropriate for both bulky and liquid output.

LARGE
Approximately 14 inches in length, larger pouches have a greater volume capacity than standard pouches, making them more useful if you have a lot of liquid output.

EXTRA-LARGE
Extra-large ostomy bags are, as it says on the tin, extra-large. These pouches are very useful if you have a high volume of liquid output, and many come with the spigot closure to make draining your pouch easier.

NIGHT POUCHES
If you find you are getting up constantly during the night to empty your bag, you may want to consider a night pouch. Although night pouches don't have the same options available regarding color, filter, etc. as regular pouches, they can hold up to 2 liters of waste and greatly reduce the number of times you'll have to empty your pouch.

CHILDREN

There are specific ostomy systems for children. Available with nearly as many options as the adult appliances, the only real difference is their tiny size and cute patterns.

REGULAR VS. EXTENDED-WEAR WAFERS

As you would expect, the main difference between regular and extended-wear skin barriers is the length of time they can be worn before needing replacement.

REGULAR-WEAR WAFERS
Regular-wear skin barriers are intended to last for three to four days

before changing.

Pros:

- If your output is more solid than liquid, wear can be extended up to five to seven days.
- There is less adhesive material on the barrier, reducing the risk that your skin will become irritated.
- Regular-wear barriers tend to be less expensive per unit.

Cons:

- Regular-wear barriers are less resistant to liquid output. If you have a lot of liquid output, you may get a shorter wear time.
- Less adhesive material means they can be more prone to peeling.
- You need to change regular-wear wafers more often.

EXTENDED-WEAR WAFERS

Extended-wear barriers are designed to last up to seven days.

Pros:

- Extended-wear barriers can last up to seven days even with
  liquid output, allowing you to change less often.
- Some types contain material that swells up around your stoma when it gets wet, creating a better seal if you have a high amount of liquid output.
- Extended-wear barriers have a greater amount of adhesive, so wafers stay attached for longer periods of time without peeling.

Cons:

- A greater amount of adhesive means you need to be more careful when removing the barrier, and more vigilant about watching for skin irritation.

- Extended-wear barriers tend to be more expensive per unit.

SPECIAL REQUIREMENTS: CONVEX PANELS AND STOMA COLLARS

CONVEX PANELS FOR RETRACTED STOMAS

A retracted stoma will be either flush with the surrounding skin or slightly sunken. Unfortunately, a concave stoma can be difficult to get a good seal around. Wafers with a convex stoma panel fill in the recessed area of the stoma and even protract it slightly, making a good seal easier to obtain.

Pros:

- A convex panel improves the barrier seal for your retracted stoma, helping to maintain your skin integrity.

Cons:

- The panels can cause bruising when used in conjunction with an over-tightened ostomy belt, or if the convexity of the wafer is too deep in relation to your stoma.

STOMA COLLARS FOR HERNIATED STOMAS

The opposite of a retracted stoma, a herniated stoma protrudes further than average. The protrusion can cause your stool to collect and "pancake" at the top of your ostomy bag, and leak into the flange. To better manage a herniated stoma, use a stoma collar or hat. Stoma collars consist of a flexible, adhesive channel that sits over your stoma and acts as a funnel to keep waste away from the flange.

Pros:

- The collars keep stool away from your flange, helping to prevent leaks.
- Collars can be used to prevent leaks even if you don't have a herniated stoma.

Cons:

- Although the collars are available in several sizes, they are
- not adjustable; you need to ensure you have the correct size for both comfort (not too tight), and efficiency (not too loose).

THE COST OF OSTOMY SUPPLIES

Another factor you need to consider when you are choosing your ostomy system is cost. When choosing an appliance, make sure you take into account whether or not you can afford that particular system for the length of time that you will have your stoma. Some systems can be quite expensive. The coverage of ostomy supplies varies between countries, with some covering all the cost and others covering none. Find out what government or private plans are available where you live. In Canada, for example, each province and territory has their own program of funding, insurance, or tax relief. Conversely, in the United Kingdom, supplies are covered by the National Health System, with a minimal prescription amount paid by the patient.

If you are not covered by a private or government program, and you are finding it difficult to afford supplies, sites like Ebay, Kijiji, and Craigslist can be excellent sources of discounted systems. Lots of healthcare stores also sell ostomy appliances online, and will often have sales or sell cheaply in bulk. Finally, your stoma nurse may have a few sources of her own, such as patients who no longer need the supplies they have stockpiled. When you are buying supplies outside of a pharmacy or healthcare store, make sure that you check the expiration date on the supplies and ensure, to the best of your ability, that they are in good condition; bags that have deteriorated or are damaged will often result in leaks.

The major ostomy appliance suppliers include ConvaTec, Hollister, and Coloplast. These companies sell their systems through both retailers and online. They also sell various accessories from other brands.

Buy the best system that you can afford, even if you would rather spend the money elsewhere. You need to view your ostomy system as a necessity; it's not worth having an appliance that doesn't work.

OSTOMY ACCESSORIES

There are numerous accessories you can get to customize your appliance and increase wear time by:

- forming a good seal around your stoma and preventing leakage
- prolonging the integrity of your wafer
- avoiding skin irritation
- treating skin irritation
- bulking up liquid output
- reducing odor

FORMING A GOOD SEAL AND PREVENTING LEAKAGE

MOLDABLE SKIN BARRIERS
Moldable skin barriers are placed around your stoma and under your wafer, allowing you to customize the stoma panel on your wafer to the exact size and shape of your stoma. A customized skin barrier will:

- help to ensure a snug fit
- provide an extra layer of protection
- fill in any gaps in the wafer, especially if you have uneven skin

Moldable skin barriers are available in the following forms:

Moldable paste (tube or moldable strips)
The paste is pulled apart in small chunks and used to fill in gaps, or you can make a ring to encircle your stoma.

Moldable rings
Moldable rings are shaped smaller or stretched larger to custom-fit around your stoma.

Moldable sheets

Sheets can be cut with scissors into ribbons, which are molded around your stoma as necessary.

OSTOMY BELT

Ostomy belts come in a variety of styles, from the purely functional to the decorative. Belts increase the security of the seal by holding your appliance snugly against your body. An ostomy belt can be especially useful if your stoma is retracted and you are using a convex wafer.

OSTOMY WRAP

An ostomy wrap is a wide band of fabric, like a tube top, worn around your waist and over your appliance. Like ostomy belts, wraps come in a range of styles, colors, and fabrics, and keep your appliance smooth and snug against your body.

STOMA COLLARS

Stoma collars are flexible plastic channels that fit over your stoma and prevent waste from pooling around the flange and causing leaks.

FLANGE EXTENDER

Flange extenders, which are available as a film or a tape, provide protection against leaks by extending the area covered by your wafer or flange and keeping the edges of your wafer from peeling. If you do get a leak, a flange extender can also work as a temporary patch until you can change your appliance.

PROLONGING THE INTEGRITY OF YOUR WAFER

ADHESIVE REMOVER

Adhesive remover dissolves any glue residue left on your skin from the previous wafer; having clean skin will help the next wafer you apply adhere more effectively.

ADHESIVE WIPES

Adhesive wipes apply an extra layer of adhesive to the skin, increase the sticking power of the wafer.

AVOIDING SKIN IRRITATION

BARRIER WIPES

Barrier wipes apply a protective film to your skin before you apply any adhesive. The thin film helps to protect your skin from the adhesive glue, preventing skin irritation and helping any injured skin to recover.

ADHESIVE REMOVER

Leftover glue fragments can chafe your skin. Adhesive remover keeps your skin free of any irritating residue.

TREATING SKIN IRRITATION

PROTECTIVE POWDER

Apply hydrocolloid powders to any broken skin around your stoma to protect it from further irritation by barrier pastes and wafer adhesive. The powder also absorbs moisture, and will help keep the skin around your stoma dry while it heals.

BULKING UP LIQUID OUTPUT

GELLING SACHETS

Placing a gelling sachet (such as ConvaTec Diamonds™ Gelling Sachets) into your pouch can magically give your liquid output a more solid form.

BULKING AGENTS

Bulking agents help absorb the digestive enzymes that irritate your skin, and can also make your output more solid. Popular types include psyllium (such as Metamucil®), methylcellulose (Citrucel®), and calcium polycarbophil (FiberCon®).

REDUCING ODOR

GELLING SACHETS
When placed in your pouch, a gelling sachet can also reduce excess gas and help prevent bag-bloat and odor.

ODOR-ELIMINATING DROPS
A few drops of deodorizing liquid (such as Hollister's m9 Odor Eliminator Spray®) in your pouch can help reduce or eliminate odor. Deodorizers are also available as a gel, lubricated or non-lubricated. Lubricated deodorizers can make your bag easier to empty by making it more slippery for thicker stool.

ROOM SPRAY
There are numerous brands and scents of room spray available. Choose one that is formulated specifically for diffusing bathroom smells (such as Poo-Pourri™), and works as a deodorizer rather than just a cover-up, which fools no one.

DEVROM® CHEWABLE TABLETS
To be eaten after a meal, Devrom® tablets (bismuth subgallate) reduce gas and odor by curtailing the odor-producing bacteria in your intestine.

The huge variety of ostomy accessories can make it difficult to choose the right ones. As with pouching systems, however, most companies are more than happy to provide you or your stoma nurse with free samples of everything they offer. Take advantage of this to try as many different products as you can. Anything you don't use, keep for emergencies or pass on to your stoma nurse or other ostomates.

CHANGES

CHANGING YOUR APPLIANCE

Although you will be shown how to change your appliance by your ostomy nurse, the following are basic step-by-step instructions, just in case you forget or are intoxicated:

1. Make sure your hands are clean.
2. Lay out everything you need. If you are using a drainable pouch, check that the outlet on the new pouch is closed. You can adjust it later.
3. If you are cutting your skin barrier to fit, measure and cut now.
4. If you are using any deodorants, gelling sachets, or liners, place in the new pouch.
5. Remove and discard your old pouch.
6. Remove your wafer if it needs to be changed.
7. Place a piece of gauze over your stoma to catch any output.
8. Remove any leftover adhesive from your peristomal skin.
9. Clean the skin around your stoma with gauze or a soft washcloth, removing any stool. Don't use soap, only warm water.
10. Ensure your skin is clean and dry.
11. Apply powder over any broken skin.
12. Apply barrier wipes and barrier adhesives as needed.
13. Apply barrier paste, rings, or strips around your stoma. If they are too warm and stick to your hands, moisten your

fingers with water. If you are using a moldable stoma panel, mold it to the shape and size of your stoma. If you are using a stoma collar under your wafer, apply it now.

14. If you are using a one-piece system, remove any gauze from your stoma.
15. Center and apply your wafer over your stoma.
16. Check to confirm you have a good seal. Adjust any molded elements. Make sure the wafer is attached to your skin smoothly, free of any folds or wrinkles.
17. If you see any gaps between your stoma and your barrier, fill with barrier paste or remove, adjust, and reapply your wafer.
18. If you are applying a two-piece system, remove the gauze from your stoma and attach your pouch to the wafer. Press the flanges together all the way around, ensuring they are securely connected.
19. Hold your hand over your wafer for 30 seconds to warm it slightly and help reinforce the seal.
20. Apply any flange extenders as necessary.

APPLIANCE CHANGE CHECKLIST

- wafer
- pouch
- measuring set: template, pen, and scissors
- pouch deodorants
- gelling sachets
- pouch liners
- accessories such as stoma bridges, collars, and flange extenders
- gauze or a soft cloth
- disposal bag
- adhesive remover
- stoma powder
- barrier wipes

- barrier adhesives
- barrier paste, strips, or rings

TIPS FOR EMPTYING AND CHANGING YOUR POUCH

You'll get taught the basic method for changing your appliance before you leave the hospital, but you may eventually need a more customized approach to deal with your stoma's quirks. Experiment with how you change your pouch and use whatever method works best for you. The following general tips will help you get started:

WHEN TO EMPTY OR CHANGE YOUR POUCH

- Empty your bag when it is 1/3 full. Any fuller and you risk leaks.
- Change your appliance promptly if you feel any skin irritation or notice any leaks.
- Only wear your appliance for as long as the manufacturer recommends. You can sometimes get away with wearing it a bit longer, but don't try to be too clever. You might be leak-free, but you may also start to smell.
- When you apply an extended-wear wafer, write the date on it in indelible marker so you don't forget when you put it on. Extended-wear wafers should be changed every seven days to help avoid skin irritation. The bag attached to it should be changed every three to four days.
- Normal-wear wafers should be changed every two to four days.
- You may need to change your wafer more often during hot weather, or if you sweat frequently. Extra moisture reduces the ability of the wafer to stick to your skin.
- Burp your bag when it is slightly ballooned; don't wait until it is turgid or lifting away from your body.

- Empty your pouch before exercising or having sex.

HOW TO EMPTY YOUR POUCH

- If you are in a public washroom and feeling self-conscious about making noise, layer some toilet paper in the water—but don't fill the bowl—or use a deodorizing powder to dampen the noise.
- If you are worried about smell, use a deodorizing spray. At home, keep a variety of scented items in the bathroom, such as candles, soaps, and sprays.
- Make sure the drainage outlet on your pouch is clean and dry before you secure it. If the Velcro® does get soiled, it's nearly impossible to clean properly, so change your bag to avoid odor and leakages.
- If you have a lot of soft, chunky output that you can't drain, remove your bag, place some gauze over your stoma and rinse the bag out. Do not rinse your bag in the toilet, because it's a *toilet*. You can also use lubricated drops to keep things slick.
- Sit on the toilet, kneel, or stand next to it; whatever method is the most comfortable for you. Open, drain, clean, seal, and go on your merry way.
- Tuck the bottom of your shirt or dress into your collar, or secure it with a clothespin; you'll avoid splash back and leave both hands free for draining your pouch.
- If you do have trouble with splash-back, try sitting backward on the toilet.
- If you're emptying your bag in a public bathroom, don't worry about the sound and smell. When are you ever going to see these people again? Besides, most people are too busy worrying about their own sounds and smell. No one will even notice you.

CHANGING YOUR POUCH

- If possible, change your bag at a time of day when you normally experience the least amount of output, such as first thing in the morning, before you eat or drink anything.
- Prepare your supplies before you start changing: cut any wafers, lay out your accessories, and check the integrity of your appliance. Keep a checklist in the bathroom to help you remember everything you need.
- Soften the adhesive and moldable parts of your appliance before you apply them by warming them in your hands for about 30 seconds. You can also warm them with a hair dryer, on the lowest heat setting, for 10-30 seconds.
- Take the time to measure your stoma if you are cutting your skin barrier to ensure it is the right size.
- Make sure your skin is clean and dry before you put on a new wafer.
- Place a piece of gauze over your stoma while you are changing your pouch to prevent any output spillage. You don't have to use gauze, but make sure whatever you do use won't disintegrate or stick when it touches your moist stoma, like tissue.
- If you have skin folds, dips, or scars that prevent you from getting a smooth adhesion of your wafer, stretch your skin as flat as possible as you put on your wafer. If you find you need more than two hands to do this, apply the wafer while you are lying on your back. To get the wafer in the correct position over your stoma, adjust the wafer while standing, then hold it in place as you lay down and smooth it over your skin.
- Position your wafer however works best for you. If a diamond works better than a square, go for it.
- Don't over-powder; your wafer won't stick.

- After your appliance is attached, hold your hand over the flange for 30 seconds. The heat from your hand will help the wafer adhere better.
- If you struggle to remove your wafer without taking off a layer of skin, soak in the tub and peel it off bit by bit.
- If you find that your barrier paste isn't made sufficiently pliable by your hands, warm it with your hairdryer on low, or put it in warm water for 1 minute before shaping.

DISPOSAL

- If you are using a closed pouch, you don't have to empty it before you dispose of it.
- Never flush your pouch down the toilet, unless it's the flushable kind.
- Dog poop bags work just as well as ostomy-specific disposal bags, and they can be purchased at more places, such as the dollar store.
- If you are using a two-piece closed pouch and don't want to throw it away each time you empty it, use a flushable pouch liner. The flange can still be sealed securely over the liner, and you will still be able to burp your bag. When you empty your pouch, just remove the liner and flush or throw away.

BREAK MY STRIDE

ODOR, LEAKS, AND OBSTRUCTIONS

ODOR

Odor is one of the biggest issues ostomates worry about, but unless your hygiene is a bit casual or you eat a lot of odor-causing foods, you shouldn't have too much trouble with it. The main source of osto-odor is when you empty your bag or burp it, and that's not much different from having a poo or a fart, is it? There are plenty of much smellier non-ostomates out there, guaranteed.

If you are concerned about odor, however, you have some options to help you control it:

GELLING SACHETS
As well as adding more solidity to liquid output, gelling sachets reduce gas and odor.

DEODORIZING POWDERS
Sprinkle deodorizing powders such as "You Go Girl®" into the toilet bowl before you empty your bag. Watch in awe as the powder forms a thick layer of foam on top of the water that muffles both the sound and any odor. Deodorizing powder also limits splash-back *and* cleans the toilet, so you'll be the perfect dinner guest.

ODOR-ELIMINATING DROPS
Available as liquid or gel, lubricated or non-lubricated, a few drops are

placed in your pouch to eliminate odor. If you have particularly thick output, lubricated drops can make your pouch more slippery and easier to drain. You will hear of various household products that you can put in your pouch to help control odor, but use them at your own risk; some of them are harmful to pouch material and can cause leaks.

ROOM SPRAY

Even self-conscious non-ostomates use room spray. Avoid a chemical porta-potty smell by choosing a spray specifically made to neutralize odor.

DEVROM® CHEWABLE TABLETS

To be eaten after a meal, Devrom® tablets can help reduce odor-causing gas.

BAKING SODA RINSE

If you wear the same bag for several days at a time, you can rinse it with a baking soda and water solution to help keep it fresh. Keep an eye on your bag's integrity, just in case.

HYDROGEN PEROXIDE

Some ostomates recommend squirting a 3% hydrogen peroxide solution into your bag if you are having issues with odor. If you try this method, and your ostomy nurse may discourage you, don't use a greater concentration than 3% or you risk your bag falling apart.

LEAKS

If you're lucky, your first indication of a leak will be the itching, burning sensation of stool leaking silently under your wafer. If you're unlucky, the drainage closure on your bag may come undone, or your pouch may split apart at the seams. If you experience any itching or burning around your stoma, check your appliance immediately. If you choose to ignore it, stool will eventually begin to seep from your appliance, and you will then feel the burning on your cheeks. Your face cheeks. Because you are embarrassed. Fortunately, most leaks occur at the flange connection or under the wafer, and can be quickly controlled if you address them straight away.

There are a number of reasons why you'll get leaks, and knowing what they are can help you avoid them.

CAUSES OF LEAKS

IMPROPER SEAL AROUND YOUR STOMA
An inadequate seal is the most common cause of leaks. A secure seal may be difficult to achieve if you have:

- a retracted stoma
- a herniated stoma
- creases or folds around your stoma
- too much powder applied around your stoma

FAILURE OF ADHESIVE
Leaks can occur under the wafer if it hasn't adhered properly to your skin because of:

- allergies or skin rashes that prevent the adhesive film from sticking
- old adhesive, soap or shampoo residue, or moisturizer film that has not been cleaned properly from your skin
- skin that is damp when the wafer is applied

- scars, creases, folds, or body hair
- barrier wipes, which can interfere with the adhesion of extended-wear wafers

POUCH FULLNESS
Your pouch may simply be too full. Your bag should be emptied when it is 1/3 full, 1/2 if you like to live dangerously.

WORN-OUT APPLIANCE
You may have been wearing your appliance for too long. Ensure you wear your system within the manufacturer's recommendations for that particular product.

HIGH-LIQUID OR VERY THICK OUTPUT
Your output may be very liquid or very thick, both of which can interfere with your seal, your flange, and your wafer.

IMPROPER FLANGE ATTACHMENT
If the flange on your system is not properly secured, it will become detached. If you are using a snap-together flange, make sure you hear it snap all the way around. If you are using an adhesive coupling, ensure it is tamped down all the way around with no air bubbles to lift the edges.

SOILED OUTLET
If the outlet of your drainable pouch is not kept clean, it will not seal properly.

CLIP FAILURE
Clips can catch on clothing or external objects and come undone.

CLOGGED FILTER
Both liquid and very thick output can saturate your filter and force stool through the opening.

EXCESS GAS

If your pouch fills with gas, it can balloon, lifting the appliance away from your skin and allowing stool to seep underneath.

PANCAKING

Thick output can gather around your stoma and push through the flange or under the wafer.

SUPPLIES ARE DAMAGED OR DETERIORATED

If your supplies have been damaged (i.e. frozen, torn, subjected to heat), or if they are past their expiration date, their integrity may be compromised, and they can simply fall apart.

SOMETIMES, LEAKS JUST HAPPEN

(I would say shit happens, but you're probably pretty tired of hearing that by now.)

TIPS FOR AVOIDING LEAKS

- Make sure that you get a good seal around your stoma. Use any necessary accessories to help you get it, and take your time.
- Once you get a good seal, leave it alone!
- If you are having trouble getting a good seal due to a retracted stoma, use a convex wafer in combination with an ostomy belt to hold your seal more securely.
- Use moldable wafers if you have an irregular stoma.
- Apply a flange extender if you have a good seal and still seem to be getting leaks.
- Ensure that your supplies are in good condition.
- If you get persistent leaks with one system, change to another. It doesn't matter if you have half a box left!
- Empty your pouch before it becomes too full. Don't say you weren't warned.
- Burp your bag as necessary to avoid blowouts from excess gas.

- If you find that stool is pancaking around your stoma, try shaking it down into the pouch to prevent it leaking into the flange. To help avoid pancaking you can use the following accessories:

  Stoma bridge: consisting of adhesive cubes, a stoma bridge is placed inside the top of your pouch to prevent stool from sticking the sides of it together and creating a backlog. If you need to improvise, wadded-up toilet paper in the bottom of your pouch can have a similar effect.

  Stoma collar: a soft plastic funnel which you can use to channel waste into your bag.

  Lubricated pouch deodorizer: a lubricated deodorizer will grease the inside of your bag and help the stool slide on down. Some ostomates use baby oil instead. If you also choose to do so, keep an eye on the integrity of your pouch since some oils can cause the material to degrade.

- Keep your drainage outlet clean and dry. An easy way is to roll up the end of the closure a few times before you empty your bag, which will help to keep the bottom edges clean. You can also wipe the mouth of the bag with a moist baby wipe or toilet paper after emptying, and then wipe dry. Keeping the drainage outlet clean can also help you avoid odor.
- Use bulking agents such as Metamucil® or applesauce to thicken your stool if your leaks are due to a high volume of liquid output.
- Make sure the area under your wafer is hair-free. Shave, use hair removal cream, wax, electrolysis, whatever. Get rid of it or your wafer won't stick.
- Empty your bag before bed to avoid nighttime leaks, or use a higher volume or night bag.
- Learn from your mistakes, and adapt.

COPING WITH LEAKS

Not only are leaks embarrassing—unless you are in a beer-smelly, darkened bar; in that case, you might as well finish your chicken wings before you worry about it—but they can also be itchy and painful. The output from your stoma is full of digestive enzymes, and it *burns*. Check your pouch as soon as you feel any itching, because even though that itch may turn out to be just garden-variety irritation, if you do have a leak, caustic waste has already started to eat your skin. Obviously, once you've discovered a leak, you need to change your whole appliance as soon as you can. It's fine to tape your system together until you can change it, but patching should only ever be a temporary measure.

TIPS FOR COPING WITH LEAKS

- Always have your kit, or a basic version of it, with you. You'll be able to sort out your leak asap if you have your supplies at hand.
- Figure out where the leak is coming from so that you can double-check this area for security when you put on your next bag.
- Use a barrier powder and barrier wipe over any red or broken skin. Your skin can degrade quickly, so take care of any irritation before it becomes an issue. Your skin takes much longer to heal than it does to damage.
- MacGyver the leak the best you can. If you don't have your survival kit, use whatever you have on hand until you can change.
- If you are having a difficult time preventing leaks, now may be a good time for you to go to the forums or blogs. Leaks are an unfortunate fact of life for ostomates, and you may be able to get some good advice and creative solutions from your peers.

OBSTRUCTIONS

You will hopefully never experience an obstruction, but you should know the signs and how to cope, just in case. Blockages can be painful and scary and, in serious cases, they can require emergency surgery to avoid bowel perforation.

CAUSES OF AN OBSTRUCTION

Blockages can be due to:

- strictures (narrowing of the intestine), caused by scar tissue
- adhesions of scar tissue
- kinks in your bowel
- ileus (the muscle of your small intestine fails to contract and move contents along)
- very high fiber foods/high risk or "caution" foods
- dehydration
- overeating
- not chewing food properly

SYMPTOMS OF AN OBSTRUCTION

Initially, a blockage may feel like painful (but benign) gas. If you have any of the following symptoms, however, you may have an obstruction:

- little or no output for several hours
- cramping and pain that comes in definite waves (due to your intestine contracting and trying to move contents through itself)
- nausea
- loss of appetite (because you already feel full and bloated)

- vomiting
- clear drainage from your stoma
- spurting output from your stoma
- swollen stoma

TREATING AN OBSTRUCTION

If the blockage is small or only a partial blockage, you may be able to resolve it yourself. If you suspect you have an obstruction forming:

- Stop eating solids.
- Drink water, coffee, tea, soda, or sports drinks; these may help to shift the blockage.
- DO NOT USE LAXATIVES.
- Make sure your stoma isn't being squashed or blocked by your appliance, or by waste pancaking in front of your stoma.
- Massage your belly.
- Rock backward and forwards, and side-to-side while on your hands and knees, or from side-to-side while on your back with your hands wrapped around your knees. Sometimes this movement will help free a partial blockage; it can also help to shift gas.
- Take a hot bath; it can relax you and may encourage movement.
- Irrigate. If you have a tendency to get partial obstructions, your ostomy nurse may show you how to irrigate your stoma. **Do not, under any circumstances, attempt an irrigation unless you have been shown how to do it properly.** You may end up with an obstruction, a perforated bowel, and possibly a Darwin Award.
- Seek medical attention. If your attempts to resolve your suspected blockage are unsuccessful, and you continue to have no output for 4-6 hours, or the pain becomes severe (you'll know), or you begin to vomit, then go to the hospital and **don't leave until your blockage is resolved.**

PREVENTING AN OBSTRUCTION

Sometimes, an obstruction will happen regardless of any effort on your behalf. Obstructions due to factors such as scar tissue, you simply can't control. Obstructions due to food, however, can usually be prevented. The best ways to avoid a blockage due to food—and yes, they are common sense, but who uses that on a regular basis?—are to:

- Avoid foods that you know are problem foods for you. (You won't literally die if you *don't* have mushrooms, will you?)
- Eat only small amounts of high-risk foods and chew them thoroughly.
- Chew ALL food well.
- Avoid overeating.
- Drink a beverage whenever you eat something.

SKIN-DEEP

SKIN CARE AND YOUR ILEOSTOMY

PERISTOMAL AND STOMAL SKIN CARE

Healthy peristomal skin is crucial to both your physical and psychological well-being. Maintaining the integrity of your skin can be a constant struggle when you have an ostomy, but there are things you can do to make it easier and more successful.

WHAT IS "NORMAL"?

- Your stoma should always be deep pink to red in color, and it should look moist and shiny.
- The surface should be relatively smooth and free of blemishes, such as granulomas.
- You should not be able to see any separation between the edges of your peristomal skin and your stoma.
- Your peristomal skin should be free of rashes, ulcers, or any inflammation, including inflamed hair follicles.

WHAT CAUSES SKIN IRRITATION?

Your peristomal skin can be irritated by a variety of sources:

LEAKS

Leaks tend to be the most common cause of peristomal skin irritation.

Your output is highly caustic and can damage your skin very quickly; when your bag leaks, those corrosive enzymes come in direct contact with your skin.

CHANGING YOUR BAG TOO OFTEN

Since cleanliness is crucial to having a healthy stoma, you may become obsessive about changing your bag. Follow the guidelines for the intended use of your product, and only change it when necessary (i.e. if the recommended time is up or if you have a leak).

TOO MUCH FUSSING

Once your bag is on and secure, leave it alone!

EXCESSIVE USE OF ALCOHOL WIPES

Not everyone's skin can tolerate alcohol wipes. Since they are not essential, you can buy alcohol-free wipes, use them sparingly, or stop altogether.

CONTACT DERMATITIS

You may develop an allergy or sensitivity to the supplies you are using. You can try using barrier wipes under your wafer to reduce the amount of contact, but you may have to switch to a different appliance.

PROLONGED MOISTURE

Your skin may be damp when you apply the wafer, or it can become damp from sweat.

A BACTERIAL OR FUNGAL INFECTION

Skin that is continually soiled and damp is vulnerable to infection.

HAIR FOLLICLE INFECTION (FOLLICULITIS)

Folliculitis under your wafer can be caused by the irritation of constantly shaving your belly hair.

DEPRESSION ULCERS

Depression ulcers are caused by pressure from ostomy belts, convex wafers, rigid two-piece systems, or too-tight clothes. Warning signs that you may be about to develop an ulcer include redness and bruising around your stoma.

STOMA GRANULOMAS

Small nodules of inflamed flesh can form on or directly around your stoma. Stoma granulomas can be caused by trauma to your stoma through extended contact with waste, injury, allergy to your appliance, rough or excessive handling, or due to pressure from your clothes. Although not harmful, they can be uncomfortable and their size and tendency to bleed can make it awkward to secure your pouch.

AVOIDING AND TREATING SKIN IRRITATION

It is important to avoid skin irritation for two main reasons. First, you expose yourself to the risk of developing an infection which can be devastating to your stoma. Secondly, there is nothing more miserable than itchy, inflamed, broken, and bleeding peristomal skin. Of everything that will have happened to you during the course of your illness, worse than the hemorrhaging, worse than the medication, worse than the surgeries, the internal infections, the blockages and bag explosions is the itching of inflamed skin. If anything will drive you mad, it's that. You may be able to handle pain, but you will not be able to handle the ungodly itching. Avoiding infection is the most important thing, but oh my god. That itching.

TIPS TO AVOID SKIN IRRITATION

GIVE YOUR SKIN A CHANCE TO BREATHE

Have a shower without your appliance. Any waste will just wash down the drain, and no, it's not gross. You can also take your bag off and sit in the bath, or even on the couch for half an hour to let your skin get some air. Try to do it at a time of day when you know your stoma will be less active, and put gauze under or over your stoma to catch any waste that does come out.

ENSURE YOUR SKIN IS DRY
Before you put on a new wafer, dry your skin by patting gently around it with gauze or a clean cloth, or very carefully, with your hairdryer on the lowest setting. Make sure your skin is completely dry before you attach the new wafer.

USE THE CORRECT SIZE OF SYSTEM FOR YOUR STOMA
One of the quickest ways to get a leak is by having a too-large flange.

ENSURE YOU HAVE A GOOD SEAL
Even if it takes you a few minutes, don't rush it. "Good enough" will come back and burn you.

CHANGE YOUR BAG OFTEN, BUT NOT TOO OFTEN
Use a combination of common sense and the manufacturer's instructions to dictate how often you change your bag.

PREVENT FRICTION ON YOUR STOMA
Granulomas caused by your appliance rubbing on your stoma may be avoided by regularly using stoma paste around the edge of your stoma. If the front of your stoma is rubbing against the pouch, lubrication wiped on the inside surface of the pouch can help prevent this.

SWITCH BRANDS IF YOU HAVE A SKIN REACTION
It may gall you to see even one pouch go to waste, but do it. It may be helpful to have several other brands on hand, just in case.

AVOID WIPES THAT CONTAIN LANOLIN OR ALCOHOL
Lanolin and alcohol are known irritants, and can cause contact dermatitis.

IMMEDIATELY CHANGE YOUR BAG IF YOU FEEL ANY IRRITATION

Try to determine the source of the irritation. If you can get away with having a peek and not disturbing your system, fine. Otherwise, take it off.

IF YOU HAVE TO SHAVE YOUR BELLY SKIN, SHAVE IN THE DIRECTION OF THE HAIR GROWTH

Consider more effective hair removal methods such as hair removal cream, waxing, or electrolysis, which can help you avoid folliculitis.

ONLY USE EXTRA ADHESIVE WHEN NECESSARY

And then, only use as much as you *need*. Don't use extra adhesive as a precautionary measure.

PREVENT YOUR POUCH FROM RUBBING

Thigh-chafing can occur with drainable pouches from both the clip and the rolled-up edges of the Velcro® closure. To prevent rubbing, rotate your appliance slightly so that the tail end is pointed more between your legs. You can also tuck the end of the pouch into an intimacy belt with a pocket, or tie a baby bib around the flange so that the soft fabric sits between the bag and your skin. Disposable cloth bibs work well; they are soft, you can throw them away if you have a leak, and they don't have a plastic backing that rustles when you walk.

TIPS FOR TREATING SKIN IRRITATION

- If your peristomal skin becomes inflamed, apply a barrier powder or paste over the broken skin before you apply your wafer. The barrier will help to prevent further inflammation, and will encourage the existing irritation to heal.
- Use a skin powder to absorb excess moisture and oil from your skin and keep it dry. Don't forget to add a sealant over the top of the powdered area, or your wafer may not stick.

- Apply a barrier wipe (on unbroken skin only) to create a thin layer of protection over your skin.
- Granulomas that are very painful or interfere with pouch security can be cauterized with silver nitrate, or in extreme cases, surgically removed.
- If you have a bacterial or fungal infection, treat it with a topical ointment and keep your skin as dry as possible. Allow the cream to soak in before applying a barrier wipe. During your infection, switch to a pouching system that requires frequent changing, since you'll have to remove it every time you apply your ointment.
- Allow your skin to breathe as much as possible, such as in the shower.
- Do not use alcohol wipes if you have broken skin, and avoid using a sealant directly on the irritated surface.
- Reduce or remove any source of pressure, such as loosening your ostomy belt or going without when you can.
- If you have only small patches of irritation, cut out pieces of your wafer over the affected patches to let your skin breathe; only do this if the size of the patches won't compromise the adhesion of the wafer.
- If you continue to struggle with your skin care, talk to your ostomy nurse. Peristomal skin irritation is something they have a lot of experience with, and they may be able to offer you some new suggestions. Your skin can become damaged quickly, so stay on top of your skin care.

SHOWERING WITH YOUR ILEOSTOMY

SHOWERING WITH YOUR BAG ON

Many ostomates worry getting their appliance wet will reduce its wear time. This can be true if you submerge it for a long time, but most pouching systems will happily weather the storm of a shower.

TIPS FOR SHOWERING WITH YOUR BAG ON

- Appliances made of fabric-feel material will take longer to dry. If you are short on time, dry your pouch with your hairdryer on its lowest setting.
- Make sure your bag is fully dry before you get dressed, or you'll end up with damp patches on your clothes and skin irritation where the closure of the bag has rubbed you raw.
- To cover your appliance and keep it dry while you shower, use saran wrap, a plastic bag, a plastic bib, or a plastic apron.
- If your bag has a filter, you must put a sticker over it. If water gets into the filter, it will become saturated and completely useless. You will find filter stickers in your box of pouches or, in a pinch, you can put tape over the filter; be careful to not tear the filter when you remove the tape.

SHOWERING WITH YOUR BAG OFF

There are some good reasons to shower without your appliance:

- It feels great.
- It gives your skin a chance to breathe.
- It gives you the opportunity to get a thorough clean around your stoma.
- It allows you to check your stoma's health at leisure, since you won't be worried about catching any output.

TIPS FOR SHOWERING WITH YOUR BAG OFF

- Run the water lightly over your stoma, rather than let it take the full brunt of the shower pressure.
- It's fine to touch your stoma to clean it; be gentle and extra-careful if you have long fingernails.
- Your stoma may bleed a bit when you touch it; this is normal.
- Clean your peristomal skin gently with gauze or a clean washcloth.
- You usually don't need to use soap to clean the skin around your stoma, but if you do, use a hypoallergenic one without perfumes or other irritants. Do not use soap on your stoma.
- If you feel squeamish that your stoma will keep cheerfully outputting waste while you shower, wear a stoma cap. It's not quite as good as a free-the-stoma shower, but it's an acceptable compromise.

SATURDAY NIGHT SPECIAL

ILEOSTOMY SURVIVAL KIT

Like with any adventure, one of the best things that you can do to cope with your new ostomy is to be prepared. That way, when accidents happen (and it is *when*, not *if*), they won't be such a big deal.

POUCH DEODORANT
Pouch deodorants are available as liquid drops, powder, or sachets. Pop some scent in your pouch and forget about it.

CHANGE OF CLOTHES
Just in case you spring a leak. Unless it's your bag closure that failed, your shirt will likely be the victim, rather than your pants.

FULL CHANGE OF APPLIANCE
If your stoma is a consistent size, pre-cut your wafer to save time. Otherwise, moldable wafers are the most convenient option.

FLANGE EXTENDER
A flange extender will increase your chances of getting a good seal and help prevent another leak.

MOIST WIPES

Unscented, hypoallergenic baby wipes work best to clean around your stoma. You can also use gauze or a soft, clean cloth, but pre-moistened disposable wipes are more convenient when you're away from home. Avoid tissue or toilet paper, or you'll be picking bits out of your stoma for weeks.

WOUND WASH

Saline wash is available in both mini bottle and aerosol form, and can be useful if you find that baby wipes don't get you as clean as you would like.

GAUZE

To put over your stoma when you change and prevent it from undoing all your good work.

PASTES, POWDERS, AND BARRIER WIPES

Any product you regularly use to attach your appliance. Some products come in pre-packaged single-use packets, so you don't have to pack an entire box. Small and travel-size versions are also a great option when available.

ANTIBACTERIAL HAND WIPES OR GEL

Essential if you can't get to a tap. Be careful not to confuse for your skin wipes.

DISPOSAL BAGS

You can buy bags specifically for ostomy disposal, but dog poop bags work just as well and, for some reason, are much cuter.

GELLING SACHETS

Very handy if your output is, or unexpectedly becomes, liquid.

BOTTLE OF WATER

Plus, electrolyte powder or a sports drink. You don't need to be out in the sun to become dehydrated.

EXTRA CLIP, OR A HEAVY ELASTIC BAND
If you are using a drainable pouch and your closure fails, an extra clip or band can provide temporary security until you can do a full change.

CLOTHESPINS
Useful to hold your shirt or dress up out of the way while you change your appliance. Don't learn this the hard way.

TAPE
Medical tape, masking tape, duct tape. It doesn't matter, although medical tape is obviously better for your skin. You can use tape to temporarily patch leaks and secure peeling wafers.

SCISSORS
If you can't pre-cut your stoma panel, you will need scissors and your stoma measuring card.

A MIRROR
If you are in a bathroom stall, you may need the increased visibility.

COTTON SWABS OR Q-TIPS®
For cleaning any particularly stubborn bits around your stoma, or for mopping away minor leaks.

FILTER STICKERS
You never know when you're going to need a shower or see Mr. Darcy swimming all by his lonesome.

MEDICATIONS
A small supply of any medications you are taking, plus any painkillers, antidiarrheals, or bulking agents.

A LIST
Detailing your medical history, current medications, and your doctor's details.

A PATTERNED SCARF

If you have a leak, you can tie the scarf around your waist until you can change. Osto-men may have risk starting a fashion trend or settle on a fanny pack.

MARSHMALLOWS

Marshmallows can slow your output down a bit in an emergency.

CHANGE

Pay toilets may be the only type available.

SURVIVAL KIT TIPS

- Have several kits if you can. Keep one at work, one in the car, one at your local pub; that way, you don't have to worry about forgetting it.
- Keep everything together in a separate, dedicated bag. Don't just fill up your purse or man-bag with items.
- Keep your kit in an easily accessible location.
- If you don't want to carry full sizes of products or buy travel-sized items, the dollar store is a great place to get various sizes of small bottles and containers.
- Rotate your supplies and discard anything past its expiry date.
- Keep anything that might spill or open in separate baggies within your kit.

FORBIDDEN FRUIT

WHAT TO PUT IN YOUR MOUTH

ILEOSTOMY DIET DOS AND DON'TS

Your diet with your ostomy can be somewhat complicated. Technically you can eat whatever you want, but you may struggle with certain diet-related issues and have to adjust your intake accordingly. Considerations for your diet while you have an ostomy will include:

- avoiding obstruction
- minimizing gas
- minimizing odor
- regulating output

Although you may find you can eat everything on the "Don'ts" list, the following is a good starting point until you adjust.

ILEOSTOMY DIET DOS

- Enjoy foods on the "Don'ts" list, just enjoy them with caution.
- Enjoy everything not on the "Don'ts" list.
- Keep a food diary, especially for the first few months. Tracking what you ate each day and how you felt is an easy way to figure out which foods work for you and which ones don't.

- Eat slowly and chew your food well.
- Drink lots of fluids to both stay hydrated and to keep things moving.
- Increase your salt intake for the first few weeks until your body adjusts.
- Continue to eat fruit; fruit such as bananas are high in potassium and can help keep you supplemented.

TIPS

- If you're constipated, drink coffee, fruit juice, or water, and eat fruit and vegetables that are either fresh or cooked.
- If you have diarrhea or otherwise high liquid output, consume bulking agents such as Metamucil® or eat foods like applesauce, bananas, peanut butter, boiled white rice, mashed potato, tapioca, toasted bread, or marshmallows.
- To reduce odor, drink cranberry, orange, or tomato juices, buttermilk, or eat yogurt or parsley.

ILEOSTOMY DIET DON'TS (OR RATHER, "DO, BUT WITH CAUTION")

Introduce the following foods back into your diet slowly, until you know how you'll cope with them:

FOODS THAT CAN CAUSE OBSTRUCTION (DUE TO BEING FIBROUS AND DIFFICULT TO DIGEST)

- fruits such as pineapple, coconut, and oranges
- fruit peels and dried fruits
- vegetables including mushrooms, celery, whole corn, raw cabbage, bean sprouts, and starchy vegetables such as water chestnuts
- vegetable peels
- nuts, popcorn, and seeds

FOODS THAT CAUSE GAS

- vegetables including cabbage, beans, onions, radishes, cauliflower, and cucumber
- milk and soy
- alcohol, especially beer
- carbonated beverages
- nuts
- chewing gum

Bonus Tip: Drinking through a straw introduces air into your gut and fills your bag like a balloon.

FOODS THAT INCREASE ODOR

- vegetables including onions, garlic, asparagus, baked beans, cabbage, and broccoli
- eggs
- peanut butter
- fish (sooooooo much odor)
- strong cheeses

FOODS THAT INCREASE OUTPUT

- raw vegetables and cooked cabbage (let's just agree to completely avoid cabbage)
- raw fruits
- dried fruits, including prunes and raisins
- alcohol
- fried and fatty foods
- whole grains
- bran cereal
- milk
- crab and lobster
- spices

TIPS

- DON'T try to be clever or daring with foods that can cause obstructions. Nothing tastes as good as an unblocked intestine feels. Exercise caution when reintroducing these foods, and avoid them if you find you have trouble. Some people can eat mushrooms with wild abandon or their weight in popcorn in a single sitting and feel no ill effects, while others can merely lick a stalk of celery and end up in the hospital. Just make sure you start with small amounts and chew everything well.
- Avoid foods you really like for a few weeks, until your body has adjusted to your stoma. Sometimes what comes out will smell exactly like it did when it went in, ensuring you will never enjoy that food again. It turns out you really can't have your cake and eat it too.

BULKING (YOUR STOOL, NOT YOUR MUSCLES)

When you have an ostomy, frequent watery stools that make you vulnerable to leaks and have you constantly needing to empty your bag, are a nightmare. While you may find eating bran cereal is enough to slow things down, adding a bulking agent to your diet can thicken your stool, reduce the frequency with which you go, and absorb some of the digestive enzymes that damage your skin. Bulking agents are also an effective and natural alternative to antidiarrheal medications.

TYPES OF BULKING AGENTS

NATURAL PSYLLIUM FIBER
Sold commercially as Metamucil®, Konsyl®, Fiberall®, Isogel®, Fybogel®, Regulan® and Hydrocil®, psyllium (also known as ispaghula) is available as powdered drinks, capsules, bars, granules, or wafers.

STERCULIA
Known as Normacol® in granular form.

INULIN
The active fiber ingredient in FiberChoice® tablets.

CELLULOSE
Sold as UniFiber, cellulose is an insoluble fiber powder.

METHYLCELLULOSE
A synthetic fiber usually sold as a powder or capsule under the name Citrucel®.

POLYCARBOPHIL CALCIUM
Sold as Fibercon® and Mitrolan®; available as a pill or chewable tablet.

TIPS FOR USING BULKING AGENTS

- Start with a single dose a day and increase as needed. Do not exceed the recommended dosage.
- Take 30 minutes before eating to maximize absorption of digestive enzymes; any later than that and you'll reduce your appetite.
- Don't overdo it: if you feel constipated, are having much less output than normal, or your output is very thick, stop bulking until your movements loosen up.
- Take your dose without the recommended extra liquid, unless you feel you've over-bulked.
- Do not take if you suspect you have a blockage.
- Stop taking if you develop side effects including itching, severe gas, stomach or abdominal pain, nausea or vomiting.
- You may find you are particularly gassy for the first few days, but this is usually temporary.

IT'S BEETS!

Given your previous brushes with intestinal and rectal bleeding, you can be forgiven for the surge of panic that rises upon the sight of a crimson-filled toilet bowl. But before you go racing off to the hospital, ask yourself, "What did I eat today?"

Like when you had a functioning colon, the color of what you put in your body influences the color of what comes out. The main difference now that you've gotten rid of that pesky colon and are passing food instead through a stoma, is that any discoloration will happen much quicker. Rather than seeing the result of those beets the next day, you may see them in a matter of hours; a much shorter time than you would expect. And in the early days when both paranoia and strange new bowel movements reign supreme, hysteria is a completely understandable reaction.

Be prepared to see carnage if you eat or drink any of the following:

- red wine
- beets
- licorice
- red Jell-O®
- tomato sauce
- any food with food coloring
- iron tablets
- spinach

BAD MEDICINE

SURVIVING HEALTHCARE PROFESSIONALS

When you have an ostomy, dealing with healthcare professionals can be frustrating. The most common issues you are likely to encounter include the following:

IGNORANCE OF YOUR CONDITION

Unless your family doctor or nurse is a specialist or has a lot of experience in gastroenterology, they will likely have only a general understanding of your condition and how best to treat it. Some general physicians may be reluctant to deal with you, and it can take days, weeks, or even months to see a specialist. You may be waiting a long time to get treatment.

You may also find that there are times when your stoma nurse, even though specially trained, may not be as adept with your situation as you are. Some nurses can become flustered if they have difficulty with your particular appliance, or if their solutions don't help. Speak up if you feel they are doing something wrong, but only after you have given them the credit they are due.

DISMISSIVENESS OF YOUR CONDITION

Dealing with even a specialist can be upsetting at times; they likely treat a number of patients whose conditions are as serious or more serious than yours, and you may feel their level of concern is disproportionate to how awful you are feeling. Whether due to perspective on their part, or just a crappy bedside manner, don't take it personally. Try to keep your situation in perspective and remember that although they can have all the theoretical training in the world, unless they've experienced your condition for themselves, they can't truly understand it from your point of view.

TIPS FOR COPING WITH HEALTHCARE PROFESSIONALS

- Keep your expectations for care within your doctor's scope. They are not psychologists (unless they are). One professional deals with one set of issues.
- Have your regular doctor recommend a course of treatment in your chart, in case you become ill in their absence.
- If your doctor has the personality and empathy of a wet fart, don't take it personally. It's tough being awesome all the time.
- If you feel that you aren't being cared for properly, speak up. You may need to find another doctor.
- Be reasonable and realistic regarding the amount and type of care you expect.
- Accept that there might not be a perfect fix; that "well" is sometimes "well enough."
- Take as much responsibility for your own care as you can.
- Express yourself in a reasonable way. Being demanding or rude will get you nowhere. Understand that, galling as it may be, your doctor holds the power, and you need them on your side.
- A perky attitude can go far in helping you to receive better care. Don't be too perky, however, or the doctor may think there's nothing wrong with you.
- If you have to cry, cry pretty.
- You doctor is more likely to be flexible with your treatment if you are confident and capable in your self-care. Make sure you

are knowledgeable, concise, and doing everything you can to keep yourself well outside of their help.

- Be willing to take advice, even if you are fairly certain it won't work for you. Your doctor or nurse will be more responsive if they feel you are trying.
- Take your medication. Yes, you may hate it or think you don't need it, but nothing will annoy a doctor more than if you refuse to follow your treatment plan and then bitch because you're not feeling well.
- If you really don't agree with your doctor's plan, then don't follow it. Sometimes you do know better. Proceed with caution, however, because you may need to justify your decisions.

NOBODY MOVE, NOBODY GET HURT

EXERCISE AND YOUR ILEOSTOMY

Unfortunately, having an ostomy is not a good enough excuse to not exercise. Exercising (annoyingly) has benefits that can be essential to coping successfully with your ostomy:

KEEPS YOUR BODY IN GOOD SHAPE
The healthier your body is, the better you'll recover and be able to cope.

PREVENTS OBESITY
Obesity can put your stoma at risk for a hernia, prolapse, and retraction.

TONES YOUR ABDOMINAL MUSCLES
Strong abdominal muscles can reduce your risk of a stoma prolapse.

GIVES YOU MORE ENERGY
And helps to reduce your fatigue.

IMPROVES YOUR SELF-ESTEEM
By giving you more control over your body.

CAN HELP BOLSTER YOUR MENTAL WELL-BEING
The more you exercise, the more cake you can eat.

REDUCES STRESS
(cake-cake, cake-cake)

AIDS DIGESTION
(caaaaaake)

KEEPS YOUR BONES STRONG
Weight-bearing exercises help to improve and maintain your bone health.

The idea of exercising with an ostomy can be daunting at first. You may feel very exposed after your surgery, and find that even simple exercise, such as walking your dog, makes you feel very vulnerable. Once you are more comfortable with your ostomy, you'll find it easier to undertake physical tasks with confidence. You might be worried about injuring your stoma—you may have nightmares about catching it on a tree branch, for example—but it's tougher than you think. There are also measures you can take to ensure you and your stoma are protected.

TIPS FOR EXERCISING WITH AN ILEOSTOMY

- Be cautious about exercising in the heat, since it will increase your risk of dehydration.
- Stay hydrated.
- Avoid any substantial exercise for at least eight weeks after surgery.
- Begin with gentle exercises such as swimming, walking, Pilates, or yoga, and build yourself up from there. Gentler exercise will help strengthen your abdominal muscles without putting pressure on your stoma.

- Avoid lifting weights that will tax your abdominal muscles for at least eight to twelve weeks after surgery. When you do start lifting again, wear a support belt to help prevent a hernia. Start with lighter weights and increase gradually.
- Don't become frustrated if your activity level is not where you want it to be. Accept that it may take longer than you think to build yourself back up. You may also have to accept that you might not reach your previous activity levels.
- Wear a support garment, such as an ostomy support belt or granny panties, to help keep your appliance secure while you exercise.
- Wear a smaller, closed pouch, so that the closure on your drainable bag won't come loose and get caught, or rub against your thighs.
- Empty your bag before you begin.
- If you are playing contact sports, wear a guard to protect your stoma from injury.
- If you are swimming, ensure you cover any pouch filters with a filter sticker or tape. Also, remember to keep an eye on your wafer; pool chemicals and salt water can wreak havoc on your wafer adhesion over time. Your safest option may be to wear a smaller, closed pouch while you are swimming, then discard it.
- If you know you're going to be sweating, apply an adhesive barrier under your wafer to improve its stickiness and wear time.

LEAVING ON A JET PLANE

TRAVEL AND SOCIAL EVENTS

TRAVEL AND YOUR ILEOSTOMY

Traveling with an ostomy can be easy, as long as you're prepared.

TIPS FOR SUCCESSFUL TRAVEL

BEFORE YOU GO

- Learn your destination's local language for directions to the bathroom.
- Get extras of any prescription medications you are taking.
- Get prescription notes for when you go through security.
- Pack double the amount of ostomy supplies you think you'll need, then pack some more. You never know if extra supplies will be available.
- Locate ostomy suppliers in the city/country that you are traveling to before you go, just in case your luggage gets lost or you run out.
- Don't scrimp or lie on your medical insurance.
- Know where the hospitals are located at your destination.
- Rejoice in the fact that squat toilets aren't a big issue for you now.

- Backpacking is much easier (although bulkier) now than when you had active disease.
- Beware that some airport security guards may be confused by the bag. Don't let them intimidate or shame you. If they're suspicious that it is filled with drugs, whip it off. Watch their reaction. Laugh.
- Download any available bathroom locater apps for the country you are visiting.

ON THE PLANE

- Bring several changes of appliance and your survival kit.
- Buy or bring your own snacks, since you never know what they'll be serving.
- Avoid any caution foods or foods that normally don't agree with you, especially if you have a long flight.
- Take your full set of prescription medications on the flight with you and put another set in your check-in luggage, in case one set gets lost.
- Put a fresh bag on just before you board the plane.
- In the airplane washroom, empty and dispose of your bag as normal.
- Take Gravol® or other dimenhydrinate travel tablets if you're anxious about flying with your ostomy; it can make you sleepy and may also slow your output.
- Bring a change of clothes, just in case you have a leak.
- Take a blanket or shawl; stay warm.
- Buy water after you go through security. Stay hydrated. An electrolyte powder or drink is also a good idea.
- If you have a long-haul flight, bring a bulking agent to reduce the numbers of times you'll need to go to the bathroom.
- Take toilet seat covers and antibacterial hand wash, since you will probably have to sit down to empty your bag and you never know what state the bathroom will be in.

IN THE CAR

- Be careful how you wear your seatbelt. The pressure of the strap over a long period can make your appliance dig into your belly, and may also shift your seal and cause a leak.
- Keep your supplies, especially your survival kit, within easy reach, just in case you have a blow-out—of your bag, not the tire.
- Empty your bag whenever you have a chance, even if there's barely anything in it.
- Map out the bathrooms en route; you'll have a better idea of how long you'll have to wait between stops.
- Limit your intake if you know you'll be traveling for a long time without the option to stop.

ONCE YOU'RE THERE

- Be adventurous with what you eat—after all, you're on holiday—but not too adventurous. Caution foods are still caution foods when you are on holiday, and an obstruction is the last thing you want in a foreign country.
- Try to avoid food poisoning at all costs. Use your judgment with street vendors, avoid buffets, and pack snacks just in case.
- Be extra careful with water hygiene, including ice cubes. Contaminated water is the easiest way to get traveler's diarrhea.
- If you are swimming in either salt water or hotel pool water, which will be filled with chemicals, keep an eye on the integrity of your wafer; salt and chemicals can wreck the adhesive and cause your wafer to peel. Either limit your time in the water to less than 20 minutes or wear a disposable pouch just for swimming.
- Keep copies of your documents on hand at all times, including a description of your ostomy, a list of your medications, your

doctor's name and phone number, and your insurance details, in case you are in an accident.

- Keep a list of serial numbers for your appliance and accessories. It will make the process of getting them much easier if you need more.
- Keep change on you at all times for pay toilets.
- Empty your bag whenever you have a chance, even if it's not full.

SOCIAL EVENTS

When you have a chronic condition, especially one that can cause a suspiciously ballooning crotch bulge, socializing may not be as straightforward as it once was. With a little foresight and planning, however, it can still be just as fun.

TIPS FOR STRESS-FREE SOCIALIZING WITH AN ILEOSTOMY

- Bring your survival kit. If your kit is large, pare it down to the bare essentials or carry travel sizes.
- Do a bathroom reconnaissance when you arrive. Know where the bathrooms are so you don't have run around frantically looking for them when you do actually need it.
- If you are at a restaurant, don't make a big production about what you can and can't eat. If you can't eat the mushrooms, fine. You don't have to order them. Nor do you have to explain to everyone WHY you can't order them; just choose something else.
- If you are having a meal at someone's house, let your host know ahead of time what you can't eat. Otherwise, you risk making them feel awkward when you can't eat what they're serving.
- Eat slow, small, and what you know. Don't take risks just because it is a special occasion.
- Don't get wasted. Being blind drunk can make it very difficult for you to empty and change your appliance properly.
- Don't talk about your illness all night. The whole point of going out is that everyone enjoys themselves. Don't ruin it by boring everyone to death. If somebody asks, fine. But keep it brief and clean.
- Always have an exit strategy. If the people you are with know about your condition, you don't need to make excuses; just tell them you don't feel well and leave. If they are unaware of

your situation, decide in advance how much (or little) you want to tell them, or just say you have a headache.

- If you have a leak while you are out, deal with it and try not to let it ruin your night. Having an accident in public can be daunting, but if you're prepared, you can sort it out quickly. Don't let the fear of accidents at any stage of your illness keep you from going out.

- Get your outfit ready the day before, plus a back-up. This way you will not be stressing at the last minute.

FIX YOU

THE EMOTIONAL IMPACT OF AN ILEOSTOMY

EMOTIONAL IMPACT OF AN ILEOSTOMY AND HOW TO COPE

Having your colon removed and a stoma created can have a significant emotional impact, even more so than your initial diagnosis. The idea of the external pouch is scary, as is the concept of permanently losing a major organ. If you didn't fully come to terms with your initial diagnosis, then the ostomy stage is where it will finally hit you; your stoma and all its requirements are impossible to ignore.

People adjust to their stoma in different ways. At one end of the spectrum are ostomates who develop post-traumatic stress, while others seamlessly integrate their ostomy into their lives without a single look back. During the adjustment period, most ostomates experience similar emotion responses.

PRE-SURGERY CONCERNS

FEAR
- You may be afraid of the risk involved with having surgery.
- You may feel fear about the outcome of the surgery and

whether or not it will be a success.

ANXIETY

- You may feel anxious about whether having surgery is the right choice for you.
- You may also worry about what your quality of life will be with an ostomy, and dealing with issues such as odor, leaks, infections and complications, injury, and the impact on your relationships and our future.

TRAUMA

- If your surgery was an emergency, you may feel the trauma of having invasive surgery that was not your choice.

EXCITEMENT

- You will probably be excited at the outcome of the surgery, which *is* supposed to make you feel better.
- You will likely look forward to being able to make plans that don't have to revolve around your illness.

POST-SURGERY CONCERNS

After your surgery, you may experience the following emotions:

NEGATIVE BODY IMAGE AND SELF-ESTEEM
Negative reactions to your stoma can include:

- Disgust and shock upon seeing your stoma.
- Embarrassment about your body's new appearance.
- Fear of what other people, especially your partner, will think about your stoma.

- Self-consciousness that your stoma may be obvious to everyone.
- Feeling that you are less attractive or desirable.

FRUSTRATION, ANGER, AND DEPRESSION

Frustration, anger, and depression can be triggered by:

- The long healing process and your slow recovery.
- Any complications which may cause a setback to your recovery.
- Your expectations not being met regarding how well you are feeling.
- Your perceived quality of care; doctors and nurses are accustomed to situations like yours and may appear to lack empathy.
- Your new limitations, and at the adjustments you have to make.

ONGOING ANXIETY

You may feel anxious about dealing daily with issues relating to odor, leaks, infections, complications, injury, the impact of your stoma on your relationships, your quality of life, and your future.

LOSS AND GRIEF

You may feel grief at:

- Losing the person you were.
- Realizing that your future will, in many ways, be different than what you planned.
- Realizing your own mortality.
- Having the surgery before you were ready to choose; the loss of choice.

REGRET

You may regret having the surgery, especially if you elected to have surgery and ended up with numerous complications.

JOY AND RELIEF

You may feel very positive about your surgery, especially if you:

- Feel so much better.
- Only realize afterward how ill you really were.
- Feel like you have a new lease on life.
- Realize that having an ostomy isn't as challenging as you thought it would be.

COPING WITH THE EMOTIONAL IMPACT OF YOUR ILEOSTOMY: METHODS, PROS, AND CONS

You may find that the strategies for coping successfully with your ostomy are similar to the methods you used when you were coping with your illness:

STOICISM

(Carry on as normal.)

Pros:
- Makes it easier for other people to deal with you and your new bag.
- Garners the admiration of your fellow man (and woman). An ostomy bag makes you look like a boss.
- If you treat your pouch like it's not a big deal, you may find that it actually isn't.

Cons:
- You may find yourself overwhelmed at unexpected times, over things you would have previously found insignificant.
- People assume that you are coping better than you actually are, and it can be difficult when you "disappoint" them.

- Others may not realize what a big deal the surgery was for you, and how strongly it has impacted your life.

TALKING TO FRIENDS AND FAMILY
(Over coffee, wine, over and over...)

Pros:
- Verbalizing your experience can be helpful and therapeutic. Many people will be curious and want to see your appliance.
- Having people understand your current limitations can make coping as an ostomate easier.
- Other people often feel reassured if they know where things stand. Discussing your operation and your daily routine can normalize the situation and make you both feel better about what's happened to you.

Cons:
- Some people just don't want to know. Many people are uncomfortable with the idea of the external bag.
- You can over-explain how your daily routine goes; most people are fine with looking at the bag, but not everyone wants to know the gory details. Let people ask questions rather than volunteering information.

RESEARCH YOUR OSTOMY
(Learn everything you could ever need to know.)

Pros:
- Being knowledgeable about your stoma can make you feel more prepared and confident; often this will help you to cope more successfully.
- Understanding your condition can help put it in perspective.
- Knowing your options can help you make informed choices about your care.

Cons:

- Learning it all can lead to obsession. You may end up spending too much time measuring your output volume and frequency when you could be out enjoying your hard-won freedom from the bathroom.

OSTOMATE FORUMS
(Lurk, post, ask, answer . . .)

Pros:

- Like when your condition was active, talking to other people in your situation can be very helpful and reassuring.
- There are lots of people out there living large with an ostomy, and they can be an excellent source of information.
- Forums are great for practical advice on all aspects of having an ostomy, especially any complications you may have.
- There is a low level of commitment required; you can drop in or out as you want.
- You can get the support you need, then put your new confidence into action.

Cons:

- Forums can present a skewed picture of living with an ostomy since many people only use the forums when they are physically or mentally in a difficult place. This disproportionate representation can make living with an ostomy seem more difficult than it is.

PERSONAL BLOGS
(An individual's account of their experience, from diagnosis to present-day.)

Pros:

- You get a comprehensive view of what life can be like with an ostomy, including the ups as well as the downs.
- Personal blogs can be a great source of inspiration.

Cons:

- Each blog represents only a single person's experience. You may want specific information that isn't covered by that particular blog.

OSTOMATE SUPPORT GROUPS
(Like Fight Club, but even more exclusive.)

Pros:

- The same as the forums, but usually with more positivity.
- It can be inspirational to see how well other people are coping.
- Support groups are a great source of practical hacks for living with an ostomy.
- The Ostomate Club is even more exclusive than the Ulcerative Colitis/Crohn's/Cancer/Diverticulitis club.
- They tend to have good food.
- Some groups will invite professionals, such as sex therapists or nutritionists, to give talks and provide support.
- If you have ostomy supplies that you're not using, meets can be a great place for swapping products.

Cons:

- There may be few ostomates where you live. However, this provides a good excuse for a road trip.
- As with any support group, there will usually be at least one person who feels (legitimately or not) that they have it worse than everyone else. And they will need to talk about it. Loudly and repeatedly, and at the expense of other members.
- If you're not coping well, any perkiness on behalf of other members can enrage you.

PROFESSIONAL HELP
(For when it all becomes too much . . .)

Pros:

- Professionals are often more equipped to help people who have been through a traumatic experience than family members or friends are.
- Therapists can help you to devise personalized coping strategies, and will prescribe you anti-depressant or anti-anxiety medications if they agree you could benefit from them.
- Your WOC nurse should be able to help you with any of the physical issues that will arise with your stoma. That's what they're there for; use them.

Cons:

- If the professional in question does not have a lot of experience with ostomates, it may be difficult for them to understand its impact on you and respond accordingly.
- Although your ostomy nurse works with ostomates regularly, they might not be as equipped to deal with your psychological needs as they are with your physical needs.
- You may feel engaging a therapist is a sign that you are not successfully coping with your ostomy, rather than the healthy coping strategy it is.
- You may become overly-reliant on professional help whenever you have a problem. You need to realize that having an ostomy is an imperfect solution that you need to be able to deal with yourself. Use your ostomy nurse as a support, not as a crutch.

PRE-OPERATIVE COUNSELING
(Meet other ostomates; meet your appliance.)

Pros:

- Speaking with an ostomy nurse and other ostomates before your surgery can make you feel less anxious. You'll see what living with an ostomy is actually like, and you may find that it's not nearly as scary or strange as you thought it was going to be. You can even practice applying and removing an ostomy appliance before your operation, which can make you more confident when the time comes for the real thing.

Cons:

- If you are really struggling with the idea of having an ostomy, this may increase your fear and anxiety.

BECOME CONFIDENT IN YOUR SELF-CARE

(Sisters and brothers, doing it for themselves.)

Pros:

- Being proactive and responsible for your own care is empowering and will make you feel prepared. If you know ahead of time what situations you may face, such as leaks or obstructions, you will have the confidence and knowledge to deal with them.

Cons:

- Don't think that you have to do everything for yourself; if you are really struggling, ask for help.

RELATIONSHIPS AND YOUR ILEOSTOMY

Like many significant physical and emotional changes, having an ostomy can have both positive and negative consequences for your relationships.

NEGATIVE EFFECTS ON YOUR RELATIONSHIPS

PEOPLE UNDERESTIMATE THE IMPACT OF YOUR OSTOMY

Since you suddenly are "cured" and no longer have your illness, some people will expect you to be the same person you were before you became ill. They can find it difficult to understand that you may still have physical limitations, and underestimate or dismiss the psychological impact that losing your colon and living with an external pouch may have on you.

PEOPLE OVERESTIMATE THE EFFECTS OF YOUR OSTOMY

If your loved ones were over-protective of you because of your condition, they likely will continue to be; they consider your stoma a vulnerability. They may still treat you like you are ill, and may question both your ability to do certain things and your own judgment of your limitations. This can be extremely frustrating, especially if you are feeling well and want to get out there and live your life. (I'm a grown-ass woman, goddamit! I can eat as much hot sauce as I want!) The coddling that you may have enjoyed while ill can get old very fast. Remedy this response by helping yourself and taking charge of your own care.

SOME PEOPLE WILL BE VERY UNCOMFORTABLE WITH YOUR OSTOMY

It is normal for people to be taken aback at first, since an ostomy is not something that everyone has seen or even knows about. Most people are uncomfortable because they are imagining themselves in your place and empathizing with you. They will eventually adjust, accept, and move on, especially if *you* treat your stoma as just another part of who you are. Unfortunately, there are also those people who will openly show disgust or other negative feelings about your ostomy based on preconceived notions about things like smell and hygiene. These people are simply ignorant asshats incapable of empathizing. Remember, this reaction says a lot more about them than it does about you, and what it says is that they're not worth having around. If someone makes you feel uncomfortable about your ostomy, don't be afraid to call them on it.

YOUR PARTNER MAY NOT BE ABLE TO ADAPT

You may continue to be more physically, emotionally, and financially dependent on your spouse than before your illness, and this continuing dependence can create tension if one or both of you were expecting your colectomy to be a miracle cure. Physical intimacy can also continue to be an issue, especially if your spouse is worried about hurting you, or is uncomfortable with your bag. While many people find that their ostomy brings a new bond of caring into their marriage, others find that their spouse simply can't cope with the external consequences of their condition.

POSITIVE EFFECTS ON YOUR RELATIONSHIPS

AN OSTOMY CAN STRENGTHEN YOUR RELATIONSHIPS

Your friends and family will be better able to understand that you are dealing with a chronic condition—no one can dispute an ostomy bag—and may find the idea easier to accept now that there is obvious evidence. It also doesn't hurt that the idea of an ostomy is pretty extreme to most people; often you'll find people have a new level of respect for what you have gone through and how well you have coped.

CHILDREN WILL RESPECT YOU

While some children feel scared about your stoma, most of them find it fascinating and even "cool". Bask in their adoration; it may be the only time in your life kids think you're cool. To them, you are science fiction personified. Enjoy it while it lasts; children are a fickle bunch.

YOUR OSTOMY CAN HELP CHILDREN LEARN TO NURTURE

Getting your children involved in your care can make them feel valued and less afraid. Let them help you set up your supplies when you change your bag, and give them small tasks, like warming your barrier strips in their hands. You may be surprised by how much they understand and want to take responsibility for, including protecting you from other people's ignorance. It may not appeal to all children, however, so allow them time to adapt if they have a negative reaction to your appliance. If they continue to be little turds about it, get new kids.

YOU CAN MAINTAIN YOUR RELATIONSHIPS PROPERLY

Chances are you will be feeling a lot better, so you can start to make up for the times you weren't well enough to do things with your friends and family. It's not that you owe them, but reaffirming your relationships will strengthen them, and can also help you with your recovery. And now that people can actually see your "condition," you may find they are more understanding when there is something you can't do.

COPING WITH THE CHANGES IN YOUR RELATIONSHIPS

- People may ask questions about your ostomy that are personal and even borderline offensive; try to find the humor in it. Most of the time, people aren't asking to make you feel uncomfortable; they are genuinely interested in learning about it.

- Accept that not everyone is going to deal well with your ostomy, and move on. It may be extremely difficult if this person is your spouse or family member, but you need to ask yourself, especially if your ostomy is permanent, whether or not you want to live every day for the rest of your life with their contempt.
- Take responsibility for your own care. The more that people can see you coping with your ostomy, the more comfortable they're going to be with it.
- Be very clear about your needs and limitations.
- Don't let your ostomy define you. The more you do, the more negative the impact will be on your relationships.
- Don't assume that you still have a monopoly on health problems; you're getting better, give someone else a turn.
- Get out there and do all the things you couldn't do when you were ill. If you wanted a new career, you might finally have the energy to make it a reality.
- Don't tippy-toe around your ostomy to make other people feel comfortable. You're the one actually living with it. That being said, don't bore people to death about it either.

POST-TRAUMATIC STRESS AND YOUR ILEOSTOMY

Only recently has post-traumatic stress been associated with illness. The term usually conjures up images of events considered far more extreme, such as combat and sexual assault. Even those people who suffer from significant illness hesitate to place their experience in a similar context; however, post-traumatic stress is becoming recognized as a very real effect of both acute and chronic illness.

CAUSE OF POST-TRAUMATIC STRESS IN OSTOMATES

THE THREAT OF DEATH OR SERIOUS INJURY
Post-traumatic stress is characterized by anxiety caused by exposure to trauma such as the threat of death or serious injury. In that context, having your colon removed and facing the prospect of either living permanently with an external bag, or having an unpredictable organ created by cutting up a perfectly healthy one, can surely be considered traumatic?

YOU CAN'T PREPARE FOR IT
Another cause of PTS in the ill is the trauma caused by a profound sense of helplessness and compounded by a lack of preparedness. In his article *How PTSD Became a Problem Far Beyond the Battlefield* (Vanity Fair, May 7, 2015), Sebastian Junger notes that highly-trained soldiers were found to have lower rates of PTS than their less prepared counterparts; there is no training to prepare you to spend your life fighting a debilitating illness.

YOUR ENTIRE LIFE CHANGES, *AGAIN*
Missing the war when it was finally over was another source of PTS addressed by Junger. It wasn't that soldiers missed the combat itself, but rather the "closeness and cooperation that danger and loss often engender." The close bonds you may have forged with others over

your disease are suddenly no longer relevant. You no longer receive the same standard of medical and familial attention, and the focus shifts away from you and the illness which has defined and influenced every aspect of your life for so long. You are no longer 'sick,' but nor are you "cured." It's easy to feel as though you have been abandoned in an uncertain No Man's Land of living one day at a time.

SYMPTOMS OF POST-TRAUMATIC STRESS

- anxiety and depression
- insomnia and nightmares
- agitation, jumpiness, and difficulty concentrating
- feeling extremely vulnerable
- guilt, shame, and self-blame
- hypervigilance about your health
- emotional numbness and disinterest
- avoidance of certain persons, places, or things that you associate to your illness
- making uncharacteristic decisions
- flashbacks or physical reactions (such as sweating, dizziness, and increased heart rate) when thinking of your surgery or defining moments in your illness
- inappropriate or overly-emotional responses, such as irritability or anger that is out of context for the situation.
- substance abuse as a coping strategy
- physical pain that doesn't respond to medication

OBSTACLES TO RECOVERY AND DIAGNOSIS

Although accepted in the medical community, a diagnosis of post-traumatic stress can be difficult to both accept and recover from. Obstacles to recovery can include the following:

GUILT AND SHAME
Some ostomates resist a diagnosis of PST because of feelings of guilt

and shame. You may feel that the seriousness of your condition in relation to others, such as those suffering from cancer or those events traditionally associated to PTS, does not warrant such a grave reaction. You may feel like a fraud or failure, as though you are asking for more attention and sympathy than you deserve. No matter how bad your condition may be, it isn't terminal. You will survive, and you may feel a certain level of guilt if you feel anything but happy and grateful.

THERE ARE SOME POSITIVE ASPECTS TO THE EXPERIENCE

About studies done on the recovery of soldiers and rape victims, Junger notes that "combat is generally less traumatic than rape but harder to recover from." This is in part, he believes, due to rape being an acute, solely horrific and traumatizing event, whereas the experience of combat is a prolonged situation interwoven with a strong sense of community and camaraderie, an experience that can be as sweet as it is bitter. This narrative can be applied to illness: pain, fear, and long recovery periods interlaced with the happiness, love, and hope of daily life.

SOCIETY BELIEVES YOU ARE LESS

Perhaps the largest obstacle to recovery from post-traumatic stress is the understanding and reaction of society. In the soldier's case, stress can result from leaving a close-knit community with common understanding, goals, and support, and reentering a culture that is comparatively individualist. In the case of ostomates, trauma can be intensified by our culture's devaluation of those who are chronically ill, especially when it comes to an invisible illness.

Contrary to public chatter, our culture is very impatient with recovery. There is a stigma towards being chronically ill or physically challenged, a shamefulness associated with dependence. As noted by S. Kelley Harrell, the sick are expected to "miraculously recover or die. That's the extent of our cultural bandwidth for chronic illness." We value the appearance of health over the individual, and as a result, there is a marked lack of understanding and empathy towards those who are chronically ill, which can result in their alienation from not only society, but from friends, families, and partners.

TIPS FOR COPING WITH POST-TRAUMATIC STRESS

* The following tips are based on personal experiences only. They are NOT a substitute for professional advice.*

Many people find that having therapy for their post-traumatic stress is crucial to their recovery. If you think you are being affected by PTS, discuss your options with your doctor.

But whether you are in therapy or not, there are lots of small ways you can cope with PTS on a daily basis:

MAKE CONNECTIONS

If you have a good support network, talk to your family and your friends. They have been there through your illness, and they may have some insight into the source of your PTS and how to help you. If talking to your family or friends isn't helpful, you may find that dedicated support groups and forums are. If you don't want to talk, you don't have to, but don't isolate yourself. Do something with someone; it doesn't matter what.

EXERCISE YOUR BODY

Many people recovering from PTS have noted how helpful physical exercise actually is. Not only can it help you feel good and make you sleep better, but it can also help you to cope with your physical reactions to the stress. And yes, dancing around your living room counts, but getting out of the house is better, even if it is only going down the street to buy a Cronut. And the best? Getting out into some good old-fashioned nature.

EXERCISE YOUR MIND

When you're doing something, live in the moment of whatever you are doing; pay attention to what is going on outside of yourself. This doesn't mean ignoring what's going on inside your head, just take time off from focusing on it. Find a new hobby that you really enjoy. It won't stop your stress from surfacing, but you may eventually find that it begins to translate into something more positive and productive.

DON'T AVOID IT
One of the best ways to deal with PTS is to be prepared; figure out what your triggers are. It may be tempting to avoid them, but facing them in a controlled way, at your choosing, can help you overcome them. Practicing breathing exercises can help you to control your response when you do trigger it. Keep a journal to track your progress. Reward yourself with another Cronut.

IT'S OKAY TO BE SAD AND ALONE
Take the time to be alone and quiet. Constantly surrounding yourself with noise will make it impossible to face what you're going through. Put on a sad song or movie, and ugly cry. Don't forget something happy for after.

USE A CRUTCH
While you are coping, it's okay to use small tricks to help you get by. Develop a mantra to repeat to yourself, or carry a talisman: anything that stimulates a sensation that you find pleasant, such as perfume, a tactile object, or a photograph. When everything starts to go tits-up, say it, smell it, lick it, whatever.

MAKE YOURSELF VISIBLE
Invite people to share your experience with you. Write a personal blog (or even a book!), contribute on forums, give talks to increase awareness about your condition, run a marathon. You will be *seen*.

POUR SOME SUGAR ON ME

SEX, PREGNANCY, AND YOUR ILEOSTOMY

SEX AND YOUR ILEOSTOMY

Sex can be a difficult thing for many ostomates. On the one hand, you are feeling better than you've felt in years. On the other, you may feel self-conscious about your stoma, especially if you are not in a long-term relationship. There are also physical issues associated with having an ostomy that may further impact your sex life.

Many ostomates find the physical experience of sex to be much more pleasant after their colectomy. They are no longer in pain, or irritated and tired from the illness and steroids, or worried about incontinence. You might not be ready to invest in a sex swing just yet, but you may finally feel more confident, and as a result, sexier.

Most partners will be so happy to be finally having sex again that they won't even notice the bag. Okay, that might be a slight exaggeration, but the point is that it won't bother them. A worthy partner will just be happy that you are feeling better and can again share a physical intimacy as well as an emotional one. You will probably be more conscious of your bag than they are.

Unfortunately, not everyone has a positive experience; some ostomate's partners don't adjust well to their having a stoma. Yes, some people are that shallow. Keep in mind that the problem lies with them. Think about how you would feel if your partner suddenly became an ostomate. Would it matter enough to you to be a deal breaker? Most reasonable people in good relationships would say no, not even close; that is likely how your partner feels. For most ostomates, the stoma is harder for them to accept than it is for their partners, who are often just happy that they and the person they love are getting parts of their life together back and making plans for the future.

Knowing what to expect can help you cope successfully with sex and your ostomy.

PHYSICAL CHANGES AND ISSUES

ERECTILE DYSFUNCTION
Some men may be unable to get an erection. A colectomy can cause minor damage to the required nerves, but most osto-men find that full power is restored within a month or two.

VAGINAL DYSFUNCTION
Osto-ladies may experience vaginal dryness and decreased feeling in their clitoris, also due to nerve damage during surgery. Vaginal sex may be painful for a few weeks, or even months, due to healing and the formation of scar tissue.

REDUCED LIBIDO
For both sexes, medication, surgery, and changing psychology may cause reduced libido, which could be temporary or permanent.

DISCOMFORT
If some sexual positions are uncomfortable, you may need to try other ones. If penetrative sex isn't an option for you in the weeks following surgery, there are other acts that you can engage in. If you're not sure what these are, Google "sex acts, list." Or ask your mom.

NO ANAL SEX

Once you've had a colectomy, anal sex is not recommended. If anal sex is an important element to your sex life, however, speak with your doctor or nurse first about whether it is advisable for you in particular, and what precautions you need to take. If you've had your rectum removed and sewn up, it's obviously not an option.

EMOTIONAL CHANGES AND ISSUES

You may:
- Wonder when to tell a prospective partner that you have an ostomy.
- Feel less confident, and worry about your desirability and attractiveness.
- Be worried about being rejected.
- Fear any associated pain, especially after years of being poked and prodded. For this same reason, you may find the idea of physical contact unpleasant.
- Just not feel sexual.
- You may worry that your partner no longer sees you in a sexual way because they have been your caretaker while you've been ill.

TIPS FOR SEX WITH AN OSTOMY

- Show your partner your bag before sex is likely to become a possibility, even if you are in a long-term relationship, so you don't have to worry about rejection or a negative reaction when the time comes.
- Wait at least six weeks before attempting penetration.
- Expect that some physical issues, such as pain or loss of libido, may last up to three months.
- Your partner's view of your sexuality in regards to your ostomy often correlates with your feelings about it, both

positive and negative. If you're feeling sexy and selling it, the chances are good that they'll be buying.

- Help yourself feel sexy. Get some lingerie, shave your legs, take off your socks; the works. It sounds superficial, but it may just make the difference.
- Wear an opaque pouch. There is a difference between your partner accepting your bag and wanting to watch it at work.
- Empty your pouch beforehand, unless you are in spontaneous throes of passion; then just enjoy it.
- Use protection; you can still get pregnant.
- Wear an ostomy cap or mini pouch, so that your bag doesn't get in the way of your acrobatics.
- Wear an intimacy belt. They are lovely and lacy and cover your pouch if you are feeling self-conscious. They look like lingerie. For osto-men, you can buy intimacy belts that look like cummerbunds. (007, at your service!) Add a bowtie for extra class.
- Pouch covers are another cute option if you want to cover your bag.
- Use lube.
- If you don't already use toys and props, now is a great time to experiment.
- Remember that sex does not have to be penetrative. Be creative.
- If you are concerned about odor, deodorize your pouch beforehand. You can also refrain from odor-causing foods prior, but this kind of planning may take some of the sexy spontaneity out of it.
- Put on a clean, fresh bag.
- Light scented candles or incense.
- If you suspect sex may be on the cards, eat marshmallows about a half-hour before to help slow down your output.
- Make sure your appliance is good and secure.
- No penetrative sex in your stoma.
- Foreplay is just as important as it was before, maybe even more so.

- Expect the first time back in the saddle to be a bit awkward.
- Don't force it; know when to quit and cuddle.
- Don't try to over-perform. It may have been awhile and you don't want to do yourself a mischief.
- Masturbate, both with or without your partner. Masturbation can help you get used to your new body, and make you feel more confident about eventually having sex.
- Try not to squish your bag, especially if it is full.
- Join an ostomate dating site; you know you'll have at least one thing in common.

WHEN TO TELL A PROSPECTIVE PARTNER ABOUT YOUR OSTOMY

Opinion is divided between ostomates about how and when to face the challenge of telling a prospective sexual partner about their ostomy bag. Some ostomates feel that being upfront and open about from the start is the best way to go, since there is less emotional investment and thus any possible rejection would less painful. Others feel that it's better to wait until the relationship is farther along before discussing their stoma, feeling that a certain level of emotion involvement will increase the chance of their partner accepting their bag without issue.

Regardless of which method they chose, most ostomates said that their ostomy bag was not the obstacle they feared it would be; most potential partners were curious rather than repulsed. In regards to those partners for whom the bag was a deal-breaker, most ostomates figured they probably had a lucky escape, even viewing their bag as a reliable douche-detector.

PREGNANCY AND YOUR ILEOSTOMY

Many ostomates worry about their chances of conceiving after surgery. Fortunately, the medical consensus is that a colectomy and stoma creation have little effect on your ability to conceive and carry a baby to term. In fact, you may even find that you are more likely to conceive and have a healthy baby than when your illness was active because you are more likely to be in good health yourself.

So, assuming that you've had the sex and conceived the baby, now what?

WHAT TO EXPECT DURING PREGNANCY

- Your stoma may change very little, or it may change a lot.
- As you gain weight and your belly begins to grow, your stoma might retract, or at the very least, become flush with your peristomal skin. This may only become an issue in your second trimester.
- Your stoma may increase in diameter.
- Your peristomal skin will become flatter and smoother, which can be a huge bonus if you've struggled to get a good seal due to creases or dips.
- If you have a Kock pouch, you may find that it's increasingly difficult to irrigate.

TIPS FOR COPING DURING PREGNANCY

- If your stoma retracts, you'll have to adjust the appliance and ostomy products you use, such as increasing the size of your flange and swapping a flat wafer for a convex one; a flange extender will further help you to get a good seal.
- A moldable wafer is ideal during pregnancy, as you can adjust your stoma panel as needed throughout each trimester. Changes in your appliance are not just to prevent leaks, but also prevent your appliance from injuring you.

- Be vigilant monitoring your peristomal skin, and treat any irritation immediately to avoid infection.
- If you experience a lot of nausea due to morning sickness, you may not feel like eating. Eat little and often, and drink meal replacement drinks if you can't keep solids down. If you find you can't keep anything down, you may have to have IV support.
- If you are vomiting a lot, you'll become dehydrated more quickly than normal; ensure you stay hydrated. Otherwise, you will need to be given intravenous fluids.
- Make sure that you are taking all the necessary vitamins, and that they are being absorbed properly.
- Avoid any foods that pose a higher risk for an obstruction. It's only for a few months!
- You may have to teach your spouse or another family member how to change your ostomy, since your stoma may disappear from sight shortly after your feet. It's possible to change your pouch while looking in the mirror, but it can be difficult to ensure you have an adequate seal.
- Wearing a two-piece system with an extended-wear wafer means you will have to try to get a good seal less often.
- You may want to begin using a larger pouch size, which will allow you to drain or change your bag less frequently.
- Later in your pregnancy, you may find that the size of your belly makes it difficult to drain your pouch into the toilet.
- Some ostomates find emptying their bags into a bowl in the sink a much easier process. Or, you may want to use a closed pouch, which will allow you to just remove and discard your bag, rather than having to drain it.
- If you are having difficulty draining your Kock pouch, use a smaller catheter and a greater amount of lubricant. It may also help you to lie on your back while irrigating. If your output is too thick for a smaller catheter, you may have to adjust your diet to include foods that encourage a more liquid stool.

WHAT TO EXPECT WHEN GIVING BIRTH

- The method by which you give birth will be based on the extent of your scar tissue. Many ostomates can give birth vaginally, but if you have a significant amount of scar tissue, you may need an episiotomy or even a Cesarean section to prevent tearing, which can be especially severe if you have extensive scarring.

TIPS FOR COPING WHEN GIVING BIRTH

- Enjoy that you don't have to worry about pooping on the table.
- Bring your own ostomy supplies to the hospital. The hospital will have appliances, but you will be more comfortable if you have the pouching system you are used to.

WHAT TO EXPECT AFTER BIRTH

- Your peristomal skin may become significantly looser, so you will need to adjust your appliance accordingly.
- Your stoma will likely shrink.
- If your stoma retracted during your pregnancy, it should begin to protrude again.
- There is a small risk that you may develop a stoma prolapse or a peristomal hernia.

TIPS FOR COPING AFTER BIRTH

- If you normally use pre-cut wafers, use moldable or cut-to-size wafers until the size of your stoma stays consistent for a couple of weeks.

BREASTFEEDING WITH AN OSTOMY

- Having an ostomy does not interfere with the production of breast milk.

- If possible, ensure that your pouch is drained before you breastfeed, since the weight and movement of your baby can make your pouch leak or disturb your seal.
- Wearing a support garment over your pouch while feeding or holding your baby will help keep your appliance secure.
- Although you should be able to hold your baby to your breast normally on the non-stoma side, you may have to lay down to offer them the other breast to avoid pressure on your stoma.

YOU CAN LEAVE YOUR HAT ON

ILEOSTOMY FASHION DOS AND DON'TS

For the most part, you can wear the same clothes you wore before you had your ostomy, especially if you're not self-conscious about your stoma. (And who has the time for that?) Just make sure you are sensible about emptying your pouch, and chances are no one will ever notice it.

ILEOSTOMY FASHION DOS

BIKINIS/GO SHIRTLESS

Many ostomates proudly display their bags. Hell, you've earned it. If you want to keep it covered, however, you can buy custom swimwear equipped with pockets into which you can tuck your bag, or you can wear a mini-pouch or ostomy cap under a normal suit. Choose a patterned fabric or a suit with ruching for further secrecy. For ostomen, carry on as normal; your regular, elasticized swim trunks are usually sufficient for coverage. Ostomy belts can be added to any kind of swimwear for extra coverage and security.

BLACK OR PATTERNED TOPS
Black and patterned top are especially useful when you are new to having a pouch: if you do spring a leak, you'll have some camouflage until you can change.

POUCH COVERS
Pouch covers are like lingerie for your ostomy bag: not necessary, but they can sure make you feel good.

TIGHT CLOTHES, WITH A COUPLE OF CAVEATS
You will need to empty and burp your bag more frequently to prevent any bulge from being noticeable. Tight clothes can also put pressure on your stoma and appliance, so if you are wearing something snug, make sure it is stretchy and not too tight. How do you know if it's too tight? You'll know.

CLOTHES WITH HIGH OR LOW WAISTBANDS
Wear any waistband that doesn't sit directly over your stoma. Be cautious with low-waisted pants, however: the closure end of your bag can work itself up and over your waistband, and may be visible if you are wearing a shorter-length shirt.

DRESSES THAT ARE TAILORED ON TOP AND FLARE AT THE WAIST
Empire waists, swing dresses, and A-line dresses flatter any figure, conceal your bag, and give you greater leeway in how often you need to empty it.

HIGH HEELS
It's not like you have to run to the bathroom anymore, is it? Unless you get a leak of course, then just Cinderella yourself outta there.

FROU-FROU UNDIES
You're still sexy as all hell, after all.

TIGHTS
Tights can help smooth and conceal your bag, and will also give you an extra level of security.

HIGH-WAISTED UNDERWEAR OR SPANX®
Granny pants will also provide security and smoothness. Buy a size or two larger than normal so they are not too tight.

MATERNITY PANTS AND ELASTIC WAISTS
This does not mean letting yourself go; there are lots of stylish maternity pants out there. Look for a pair with a wide, soft, lovely, high cotton panel. The panel keeps everything tucked in and makes your muscles feel more supported, which is comforting if you've just had surgery. Sweatpants are another comfortable choice, just keep it on the right side of stylish. There are a lot of options that look as good as they feel.

SHORT-SHORTS
Opt for a small to medium-sized bag, however, so you don't look like your rude bits are hanging out.

A SUN HAT
If you're going to be out in the sun for a long period, a sun hat will help stave off dehydration.

AN INTIMACY BELT AS LINGERIE
You can get some beautiful lacy ones that compliment all your bare essentials.

ANYTHING WITH PLEATS
It's an optical illusion! Pleats create curves to complement your pouch.

A MODERATELY SNUG TANK TOP UNDER YOUR SHIRT
Tank tops help keep your appliance smooth and secure and also prevent it from catching on any fastenings.

A T-SHIRT EXTENDER

A wide band of fabric worn over your appliance that extends over the top of your pants like a faux top to protect your modesty.

BONUS TIP:

If you have a bag bulge but can't make it to the bathroom quite yet, tie a scarf around your waist. This trick also works for leaks.

ILEOSTOMY FASHION DON'TS

VERY TIGHT CLOTHES

Unless it is for a short time, and you empty your bag frequently. Otherwise, you may look like you have an awkward erection/lady boner, and the pressure may make your stoma uncomfortable.

WHITE

You actually can, but be vigilant for leaks.

A TIGHT WAIST THAT CUTS ACROSS YOUR STOMA

Too much pressure can injure your stoma and also restrict its function.

BAGGY, SHAPELESS CLOTHING

Unless that's what you were wearing before your ostomy.

THIN, CLINGY FABRICS

They cling to every little line and bump and can make you self-conscious even if you *don't* have a stoma.

BONUS TIP:

If you are drinking alcohol, avoid wearing a long dress, a playsuit, or anything tricky to keep up and out of the way while you are emptying your bag.

I'M WITH STUPID

ILEOSTOMIES FOR DUMMIES

ILEOSTOMIES FOR DUMMIES: TRUE OR FALSE

Most people have only a vague idea of what it means to have an ostomy. Consequently, there are many urban legends and preconceived notions about the reality of life as an ostomate, some understandable and some completely bizarre. Assumptions people make when you have an ostomy can include the following:

THAT YOU HAVE A BIG LOOP OF INTESTINE HANGING OUTSIDE YOUR BODY
False. You have a small end-bit sticking out, not a massive sausage coil.

THAT EVERYONE CAN TELL/SEE IT
False. Ostomates are like ninja cats. People will usually only know if you tell them, or if you're naked . . . and sometimes not even then. Because, boobs.

THAT IT IS PERMANENT
Sometimes true, sometimes false. The average person does not know much about ostomies; they know even less about the existence of j-pouches.

THAT YOU CAN NEVER GO SWIMMING AGAIN
False. You can even swim without your bag on. Contrary to popular belief, the water will not go up your stoma.

THAT YOU SMELL
Possibly true, but it's usually nothing to do with your stoma.

THAT YOU HAVE TO EAT BABY FOOD
False. You do not have to completely change your diet when you have an ostomy. Most ostomates find they can eat the same foods (or an even greater variety) as before their ostomy.

THAT YOU MUST HAVE HAD CANCER
False. This idea is becoming less prevalent as inflammatory bowel disease is more publicly discussed.

ONLY ELDERLY PEOPLE HAVE OSTOMIES
False. Most people associate an ostomy as a result of bowel cancer, which occurs mainly in older people.

THAT YOU CAN'T BE SMOKING HOT
False. All you have to do is look in the mirror and you *know* you're still a hottie.

THAT YOU ARE UNATTRACTIVE TO PROSPECTIVE PARTNERS
False. You may be unattractive to *certain* prospective partners, but either they're complete asshats or it has nothing to do with your stoma.

THAT YOU ARE OR WILL ALWAYS BE ALONE
False. Although after all the poking, prodding, and stupid questions, there will be times when you probably *wish* that you were.

THAT YOUR RELATIONSHIP WITH YOUR PARTNER MUST BE FRAUGHT WITH ISSUES
Quite possibly true , but those issues are not necessarily about your

stoma.

THAT YOU CAN'T HAVE A SEX LIFE

False. In fact, you have a new accessory for your sexy dance routine.

THAT YOU CAN HAVE SEX IN YOUR STOMA

False. No. No. No. Why? No.

THAT YOU CAN'T HAVE A NORMAL PREGNANCY

False. You may need a bit more help to change your pouch once it disappears from view, but at least you don't have to worry about hemorrhoids!

THAT YOU ARE DISABLED

True. But not necessarily in the way that people think of as "disabled."

THAT YOU ARE COMPLETELY WELL

False. Ostomates have their own set of trials and tribulations.

THAT YOU HAVE A LOW QUALITY OF LIFE

False . At times, you will, but your overall quality of life is likely a lot better than it was when you had active disease.

THAT YOU HAVE A POOR PROGNOSIS

False. Your prognosis is excellent—much better than it was when you were ill.

THAT YOU HAVE TO WEAR SPECIAL CLOTHES

False. You can wear special clothes, but you don't have to. Although, sometimes it's nice to get dressed up for dinner.

THAT YOU HAVE A "BARBIE BUTT"

False. Some permanent ostomates do in fact have their rectums closed, but it is not a mandatory part of having an ostomy.

THAT YOU MUST BE UNHEALTHY

False. Many ostomates find they are much healthier once they've had their colons removed.

THAT YOU MUST HAVE BEEN FAT

False. No idea where this one comes from; a colectomy is not normally a method of weight-loss surgery.

THAT YOUR COLON WILL GROW BACK

False. Although if it does, you've got your ticket to join the X-Men.

THAT ALL OSTOMIES ARE THE SAME

False. There are colostomies, ileostomies, and urostomies.

THAT YOU POO EVERYWHERE

False. Obviously, you're not just walking around with your stoma uncovered. Although it *is* a lot easier to create flaming door-step poop-bags now. Who needs a dog?

THAT THEY KNOW WHAT YOU'RE TALKING ABOUT

Depends. If they are smiling and nodding, the answer is probably false.

THAT YOU HATE IT

Hopefully false. That stoma allows you to be relatively disease-free and probably improved your quality of life. It's not a perfect solution, but it's the best one you've got.

THAT YOU ARE 100% ACCEPTING OF IT

False. Although you know it improved your quality of life, that doesn't mean you love it or are completely okay with it.

THAT YOU LITERALLY WEAR A BAG

False. Contrary to some beliefs, companies actually make bags just for ostomies, allowing you to re-use your shopping bags for something else.

THAT IT'S UNCOMMON

False. True, they're not as common as general ignorance, but everyone probably knows at least someone who has an ostomy; they may just not know it.

THAT IT IS VERY DIFFICULT TO CARE FOR

False. Unless you have a problem stoma, once you get the hang of it, your stoma care is generally straightforward.

THAT YOU ARE CONSTANTLY IN PAIN

False. There will be times when you are in pain, but since there are no sensory nerve endings in your stoma, the sheer fact of its existence doesn't cause you pain.

THAT YOU CAN'T PLAY SPORTS

False. Strap on a stoma guard and you're good to go.

THAT YOU ALSO PEE AND MENSTRUATE THROUGH YOUR STOMA

False. Somebody was smoking behind the bike shed during biology.

THAT YOU WOULD BE BETTER OFF DEAD

False. What? And miss all that good shit on Netflix?

FAKE PLASTIC TREES

SOCIAL MEDIA

SOCIAL MEDIA DOS & DON'TS

Thanks to social media, you can now tell people how you're feeling the minute you feel it. But just because you can, doesn't mean you should. Posting about your illness when you have a chronic condition like an ostomy can be tricky, especially if you have a tendency to post mainly negative comments. Occasionally telling everyone how awful you feel can be comforting as a way to both vent and get some well-deserved love thrown back your way, but constant status reports on just how hard you have it does both yourself and friends a disservice. Social media was not created with the sole purpose of providing you with a captive audience for a blow-by-blow account of the trials of your life.

Consider how you view posts on social media. Do you have a friend whose feed consists in large part of complaining about how crappy their life is? Even if their bitching is perfectly justified, after the first few posts and your sympathetic responses, chances are you have begun to dread seeing their name appear on your feed. You may feel resentful at the constant and obvious expectation for you to respond to what seems less like a sharing of feelings and more like an invitation to a self-indulgent pity-party. Since nothing you say seems to make a difference anyway, the whole exercise becomes tiresome, and you struggle to sympathize. Be honest; if you're not already ignoring that person's posts, you're probably considering it. If you don't feel this way, then you're either a saint or lying. And who could blame you? You have your own crap to worry about.

Whether this reaction to another person's hardships is right or wrong is not the point; it's simply how the majority of people feel. While people are happy to extend kindness and compassion to someone they like or love, they also have an understandable desire to carry their own burdens. I'm not saying you shouldn't discuss your illness on social media; you should. But talk about it in a way that is inclusive rather than alienating, and you'll find that people are more than happy to give you the support you need.

DOS

BE POSITIVE
Although it can be difficult at times, try to post comments about your illness only if they are positive. Positive posts can include personal milestones you've reached, good news you've received, or goals you've achieved in spite of your illness.

BE EDUCATIONAL
Bring awareness to your illness as a whole, rather than just your personal experience of it, by posting relevant articles about topics such as new breakthroughs in treatments. People who are genuinely curious will have a look, and those who aren't can bypass them.

BE FUNNY
Humor is often the best way to let people know how you are feeling without seeming as though you want pity. People enjoy laughing, and having a stoma is a goldmine for universally enjoyed potty humor. That said, keep it clever and classy; otherwise people just think you're crude.

BE HONEST
At the end of the day, be honest with yourself. You are posting about your illness because you want attention and sympathy. That is not a bad thing; you deserve it. But do it sparingly and in a way in which people feel they can be supportive without being obligated to carry

you.

BE PART OF A GROUP
There are social media groups for people ostomies. If you need to vent, vent to people who can properly empathize. You may not be special, but you'll be understood.

BE REALISTIC
Don't post with the sole intention of seeing how many of your friends respond and then measuring your worth against these responses, or lack thereof. Social media is used by people to socialize with minimal effort on their part. Understand it as such.

DON'TS

BE SELF-PITYING
Nothing scatters people to the wind like self-pity. Self-deprecation is fine, but self-pity makes people very uncomfortable. You'll get supportive comments back from some people, but many will eventually steer clear of you. Fair? Maybe not, but it's reality.

BE ANGRY
Like self-pity, anger about your condition makes people very uncomfortable. It's no one's fault that you are ill, not even your own. The universe doesn't give a shit, so there's no point raving about it.

BE SELF-ABSORBED
Even if you are posting positive comments about your illness, do so judiciously. People get bored of seeing that crap constantly infiltrating their timelines. You're ill. We get it!

TAKE SELFIES IN THE HOSPITAL
Thumbs up after a successful surgery? Good. Pouty face in hospital bed that screams "I need even MORE attention than 24-hour medical care can provide"? Bad.

TRY TO BAIT SYMPATHY

Read your post aloud before you send it. It can be painfully obvious that you are fishing for attention when you think you're being easy-breezy.

TAKE IT PERSONALLY

People have their own lives to live and are usually more concerned with that than how many bowel movements you've had today. It's not that they don't care, it's . . . Well, it's that they don't care. It's not personal; it's cat videos.

WHEN UNDER ETHER

A GUIDE TO BEING IN THE HOSPITAL

HOSPITAL SURVIVAL KIT

YOUR OWN PAJAMAS

Having your own PJs makes a difference both physically and psychologically. It's far more pleasant to be lying there in something soft and beautiful you've picked, rather than an over-starched burlap bag that a hundred people have worn. If morphine makes you adventurous, definitely opt for pajama pants to guarantee your ass is covered.

WIPES

Although hospitals do have toilet paper, it ain't the good stuff. Plus, you can use the wipes for your hands, your face, etc. if you won't be getting out of bed for a while.

YOUR OWN COFFEE CUP

Make yourself at home.

PEN AND PAPER

Just think about how many classics have been written while the authors have been off their tits in a drug-fueled haze. See this as your opportunity.

COMPUTER

Load it up with movies, TV, games, whatever. Try to make everything available offline, because some hospitals charge for internet usage. If you can then get your eyes to focus, you're golden. If you really want to be online, but don't want to pay, bring mobile WiFi.

BOOKS, MAGAZINES, ETC.

Magazines are especially good since there is usually a roaring trade of swapsies. Don't bring anything too intellectual, however; due to the morphine, chances are you won't remember anything you've read.

SLIPPERS

Most hospitals are pretty clean. But still. Slippers can be especially useful in a surgical or GI ward since there is sometimes blood and other accidents. Get the non-slippery kind.

MIRROR, TWEEZERS, MANICURE SET

Being in the hospital may be the only time you get to pamper yourself, so take advantage.

HAIRBRUSH AND HAIR ACCESSORIES

It's purely psychological. Plus, single doctors and nurses.

SOAP, SHAMPOO, AND YOUR OWN TOWEL

You can get this stuff from the hospital, but your own is so much better.

BATHROBE AND SHOWER SHOES

Trying to get dressed again in a wet shower room is the *worst*.

MENSTRUAL PADS

Yes, the hospital does supply menstrual pads, but unless you enjoy wedging a comically large brick of cotton between your legs, bring your own.

YOUR TEDDY
Just make sure you wash it when you get home.

PHOTOS
Photos of your family serve as a memento of what you have to look forward to when you get out. This reminder can help make your hospital stay more bearable, especially if you can't stand some of them.

A HOBBY OF SOME KIND
You never know how long you may be in the hospital. I became a cross-stitch adept due to the amount of time I spent inside.

MOISTURIZER
For some reason, hospitals are really damn dry.

MONEY
For bribes and for the mobile snack cart that delivers bedside.

OSTOMY SUPPLIES
If you already have an ostomy, pack plenty of your own supplies. The hospital will have a ready supply, but you'll cope better with a familiar appliance.

RULES OF HOSPITAL ETIQUETTE

YOU ARE NOT STAYING AT A HOTEL
Before you complain about the food, the 'service,' or even the lighting, stop and think about where you are. If you're well enough to complain about everything, you're well enough to go home.

NURSES ARE NOT SERVANTS
I understand that the uniforms are confusing. I know that you're scared, and you're sick, and you're in pain. So am I. And yet, I don't feel that it gives me the right to be an asshole. If you can haul yourself out of bed and down the hall to have a cigarette, don't soil the bed because it is "the nurse's job" to wipe your butt. Have some respect.

SHUT UP
I'm avoiding eye contact with you for a reason. The curtain is drawn around my bed for a reason. I'm pretending I'm dead *for a reason*. That reason is that I don't want to talk to you. If you just wanted to say "Hi," great, "Hello!" But you don't. You want to tell me your life story, and you want to hear mine, and I am sorry, but I am just not interested. My sympathy well has run dry. I am tired, and in pain, and I just want to watch *Game of Thrones*.

HAVING SEX IS NOT APPROPRIATE
Ever.

TAKE YOUR MEDICATION
Nobody is going to give you a gold star for being tough and not taking your pain meds, but I *will* punch you in the teeth when you start whining, because you're what? In pain? Also, NOBODY LIKES HEPARIN. But you'll like a thrombosis even less, I promise.

DON'T BE MELODRAMATIC
People may die right in front of you. It's sad, and scary, and awful. Don't you dare make it about you and your feelings, *especially* when their loved ones are there.

WASH

If you can't make it to the shower on your own, get the nurses to help you. I understand that we're all a bit stinky on the GI and surgery wards, but there's a limit. I inadvertently laid in my own filth for two days while temporarily paralyzed after my first surgery, and neither the nurses nor I noticed the smell because the woman in the bed next to mine had refused to wash for *days*.

YOU ARE NOT THE ONLY PATIENT ON THE WARD

You may be on a ward with patients whose illness is more serious than yours. (Hard to imagine, I know.) Make your needs clear, but not every five minutes. The nurses will get to you as soon as they can, if for no better reason than to shut you the hell up.

DO NOT MAKE YOURSELF UP AND SPEND YOUR TIME TAKING POUTY SELFIES

This makes you look like an asshole at any time, but *especially* at this time.

A "THANK YOU" BASKET FOR THE NURSES AFTER YOUR STAY WOULDN'T GO AMISS

And not a crappy fruit basket either.

HOW TO ENJOY YOUR STAY

TRY TO THINK OF IT AS A HOLIDAY
You are encouraged to take free narcotics; you get to choose your meals from a menu and have them delivered to your bedside; your linen is changed daily; you can sleep whenever you want. It may not be the best holiday you've ever had, but you did pay for it in blood, tears, and taxes, right? You might as well enjoy it.

UNDERSTAND THE SYSTEM
Stock up on breakfast items. Breakfast tends to be the best meal of the day. After that, things can get weird. Fill the drawer in your little nightstand with as many peanut butter packets and bananas as you can, even if you hate bananas.

BEHOLD THE MYSTERIOUS TAPESTRY OF HUMAN LIFE
Some of the strangest shit you will ever experience will be in the hospital. Roll with it. If a lady thinks you're her husband and tries to get into bed with you, choose to think it's because her husband has fabulous, perky breasts and not because you have a steroid beard. Don't take it personally if she later tries to stab you with a butter knife.

IT'S HOBBY TIME!
You finally have some free time to enjoy your hobbies. Knit, make lists, or finish Skyrim.

BINGE WATCH/READ
Catch up on every book, TV show, or movie you always wanted to enjoy.

WRITE LETTERS
Having to look your mortality in the face may make you re-evaluate your life. Write letters to people telling them the things that you have always wanted to tell them. Especially if you want to tell them you

think they're an asshole. They need to know, and you may not get another chance.

YOU HAVE NO CHORES
Except eat, maybe walk a few steps, and keep yourself clean. Easy.

YOU HAVE AN ADJUSTABLE BED
Up, down, slanty, flat; lots of people would kill to have one of these at home.

YOU'LL GET SYMPATHY GIFTS
Everyone who visits you in the hospital feels they should bring gifts, unless they're horrible. Yes, you will probably get a lot of grapes, but you'll get some good stuff too, I promise.

PRACTICE PASSIVE-AGGRESSION
If you're not fond of the person who is visiting, you can always pretend to fall asleep. Stare into space for a few seconds, mumble "Thank you so much for coming to see me . . . " and down you go.

CLOSE YOUR CURTAIN
Enjoy the peace and quiet.

BOND WITH YOUR FAMILY MEMBERS
Get your significant other to become your shower boy/girl. They'll get to feel helpful, and you'll get to be scrubbed down by someone who has already seen you naked. Try not to look too sexy (see Rules of Hospital Etiquette).

MAKE FRIENDS, OR NOT
You can meet some very nice, interesting people in the hospital, especially if you share a condition. At the same time, don't feel that you have to be social with anyone. Just focus on getting yourself ready for the rest of your life.

CAN'T KEEP JOHNNY DOWN

TOUGH LOVE RULES FOR SURVIVING YOUR ILEOSTOMY

IT IS OKAY TO FEEL SORRY FOR YOURSELF, BUT DON'T BE OBNOXIOUS ABOUT IT
Self-pity is destructive and even worse, boring.

SYMPATHY IS FICKLE
Don't milk it.

BE PROACTIVE IN CARING FOR YOURSELF
Choosing not to accept your condition and be proactive about caring for yourself is a self-indulgence that will make you, and everyone around you, miserable.

ACCEPT HELP WHEN IT IS OFFERED, BUT HELP YOURSELF WHENEVER YOU CAN
Develop a good relationship with your stoma nurse, but do not become dependent on them.

BE SELFISH WHEN YOU *NEED* TO BE
This does not mean all the time.

USE A COMBINATION OF COPING STRATEGIES
Do what works for you, not what other people tell you that you should be doing.

REALIZE YOUR STOMA IS NOT A PERFECT SOLUTION
Living with an ostomy is an ongoing process; you will have setbacks. Move on.

DON'T BE A MARTYR
Remember Total Recall? Quaaaaaaaaaid? It could be much worse.

DON'T BE A LONE WOLF
There are lots of ostomates and great personal blogs out there about living with an ostomy; use them.

MAKE FRIENDS WITH YOUR STOMA
Touch it, give it a name. Remember, it saved your life.

GET OVER ANY REGRETS
Most (if not all) surgeons would not have removed your colon unless they thought it was necessary or inevitable. Why regret something you had no choice about?

ALLOW YOURSELF TO GRIEVE
Briefly. Then move forward.

SCARS ARE AWESOME
You only get them if you survive something.

KEEP A DIARY OR WRITE A BLOG
You'll be able to look back and see how far you've come.

MAINTAIN GOOD HYGIENE
Don't continue to support preconceived notions about ostomy bags and ruin it for the rest of the ostomates.

DON'T LET YOUR OSTOMY DEFINE YOU
The more you do, the more negative the impact will be on your recovery, quality of life, and your relationships.

YOU ARE MUCH MORE BOTHERED ABOUT THE WAY YOUR BODY LOOKS/SOUNDS/SMELLS THAN ANYONE ELSE IS
Really.

FORCE YOURSELF TO GO OUT
You will probably have fun. Also, if you don't, people will eventually stop asking.

REMEMBER:
If you're not feeling even a tiny bit of illness, pain, nausea, sadness, anger, fatigue, irritation, itchiness . . .

IT'S BECAUSE YOU'RE DEAD.

ACKNOWLEDGEMENTS

Much love to my family and friends for their support: my time with my ostomy was both the most difficult and the most surreal part of my journey.

Jamie, you never once saw me as less than the woman you married; you have always made it so easy for me to become more.

Extra thanks to Val Cross and Julie McBride for their critique and advice: any improvements were yours. And to Mia Darien, thank you for taking on my project without a second thought.

And finally, to my surgeons: Thank you for giving me a good one.

APPENDIX
SURVIVAL KIT CHECKLISTS

*For printable checklists, go to screamingmeemie.com

ILEOSTOMY SURVIVAL KIT CHECKLIST

- ☐ pouch deodorant
- ☐ change of clothes
- ☐ full change of appliance
- ☐ flange extender
- ☐ moist wipes
- ☐ wound wash
- ☐ gauze
- ☐ pastes, powders, and barrier wipes
- ☐ antibacterial hand wipes or gel
- ☐ disposal bags
- ☐ gelling sachets
- ☐ bottle of water
- ☐ extra clip, or a heavy elastic band
- ☐ clothespins
- ☐ tape
- ☐ scissors
- ☐ a mirror
- ☐ cotton swabs or Q-tips®
- ☐ filter stickers
- ☐ medications
- ☐ a list
- ☐ a patterned scarf
- ☐ marshmallows
- ☐ change

APPLIANCE CHANGE CHECKLIST

- ☐ wafer
- ☐ pouch
- ☐ measuring set: template, pen, and scissors
- ☐ pouch deodorants
- ☐ gelling sachets
- ☐ pouch liners
- ☐ accessories such as stoma bridges, collars, and flange extenders
- ☐ gauze or a soft cloth
- ☐ disposal bag
- ☐ adhesive remover
- ☐ stoma powder
- ☐ barrier wipes
- ☐ barrier adhesives
- ☐ barrier paste, strips, or rings

HOSPITAL SURVIVAL KIT CHECKLIST

- ☐ pajamas
- ☐ wipes
- ☐ coffee cup
- ☐ pen and paper
- ☐ computer
- ☐ books and magazines
- ☐ slippers
- ☐ mirror, tweezers, and manicure set
- ☐ hairbrush and accessories
- ☐ soap
- ☐ shampoo
- ☐ towel
- ☐ bathrobe
- ☐ shower shoes
- ☐ menstrual pads
- ☐ teddy
- ☐ photos
- ☐ hobby supplies
- ☐ moisturizer
- ☐ money
- ☐ ostomy supplies

GLOSSARY

appliance: Your external waste collection device; or 'ostomy bag'. It normally consists of an adhesive wafer and bag placed over your stoma.

burping: Open your pouch at the flange attachment to release excess gas. Essentially manual farting.

colostomy: An opening surgically created to bring part of your large intestine through the surface of your abdomen to form your stoma. You may have an ascending, transverse, descending, or sigmoid colostomy, and it may be temporary or permanent.

endostomy: When the end of the ileum (small intestine) is used to form a single stoma. Can be permanent or temporary.

ileostomy: An opening surgically created to bring your small intestine through the surface of your abdomen to form your stoma. You will have either an endostomy or a loop ostomy, and it may be temporary or permanent.

loop ostomy: A loop of your small bowel is used to form your stoma, resulting in two openings. This type of ostomy is usually temporary, and always annoying.

obstruction: A blockage in your small intestine that prevents you from outputting waste

ostomate: A person with an ostomy (i.e. you)

ostomy: An opening in the body that has been surgically created to allow the discharge of bodily waste.

output: The waste that passes through the stoma. Non-ostomates call it poo.

peristomal skin: The skin around your stoma. Maintaining its integrity will become a focal point for your existence.

pouch: A more casual term for your appliance.

stoma: The open end of your intestine that protrudes outside of your body, and through which your waste is passed.

INDEX

A

access to public bathrooms, 13
    Can't Wait, **13**
    GoHere, 13
    RADAR key, 13
    Washroom Finder, 13
adhesive remover, 31, 32
adhesive wipes, 32
advantages of an ileostomy, 4–5
avoiding skin irritation, 32

B

B12 deficiency, **8**
bag. *See* pouch
barrier wipes, 32
bulking agents, 32, 67-68
bulking up liquid output, 32
bulking your stool, **67–68**

C

Can't Wait, **13**
changing your appliance, **35–40**
    changing your pouch, **39–40**
    checklist, 36–37
    disposal, 40
    how to empty your pouch, 38-39
    step-by-step, 35–36
    when to empty or change your
        appliance, 37–38
choosing your appliance, **15–28**

children, 25
closed vs drainable, 18–20
cost, 29
filtered vs non-filtered, 21–22
herniated stomas, 27–28
one-piece vs two-piece, 17–18
pre-cut vs cut-to-fit vs moldable, 22–
    24
regular vs extended-wear, 26–27
retracted stomas, 27
size, 24–25
translucent vs opaque, 20–21

D

dehydration, 8, 48, 76, 115
Devrom® tablets, 33, 42
diet, **63–66**
    diet don'ts, 64–66
    diet dos, 63–64
disadvantages of an ileostomy, 3–4

E

emotional impact of an ileostomy, **85–
93**
    coping: methods, pros, and cons, 88–
    93
    post-surgery concerns, 86–88
    pre-surgery concerns, 85–86
exercise, **75–77**

mucus, 8

N

nausea, 8

necrotic stoma, 9

O

obstructions, **48–50**

  causes of, 48

  prevention of, 50

  symptoms of, **48–49**

  treatment of, 49–50

odor, **41–42**

odor-eliminating drops, 33, 41

ostomy accessories, **30–33**

  adhesive remover, 31, 32

  adhesive wipes, 32

  barrier wipes, 32

  bulking agents, 32

  Devrom® chewable tablets, 33

  flange extenders, 31

  gelling sachets, 32, 33

  moldable skin barriers, 30–31

  odor-eliminating drops, 33

  ostomy belt, 31

  ostomy wrap, 31

  protective powder, 32

  room spray, 33

  stoma collars, 31

  treating skin irritation, 32

ostomy belt, 31

ostomy supplies. *See* choosing your

  appliance

ostomy wrap, 31

P

pain, 7,

phantom rectum, 8, 12

physical consequences of an ileostomy,

  7–12

post-traumatic stress, **98–102**

pouch, 16

pregnancy and your ileostomy, **108–11**

  after birth, 110

  breastfeeding, 110–11

  during pregnancy, 108–9

  giving birth, 110

prolonging the integrity of your wafer,

  31-32

R

RADAR key, 13

reducing odor, 33

relationships and your ileostomy, **94–97**

S

sex and your ileostomy, **103–7**

showering with your ileostomy, 57-58

skin barrier, 22-23

skin care, **51–56**

  avoiding skin irritation, 53–55

  causes of irritation, 51–53

  treating skin irritation, 55–56

  what is normal, 51

skin irritation, 8, 32, **51-56**, *See* skin care

social events, **83–84**

social media and your ileostomy, **123–26**

stoma collars, 31

stoma prolapse, 9

stoma retraction, 10

stoma trauma, 10

stool discoloration, 69

survival kits, **59-62**, **127-29**

  hospital survival kit, 127–29

ileostomy survival kit, 59–62

CPSIA information can be obtained
at www.ICGtesting.com
Printed in the USA
LVHW030235241220
674974LV00003B/429